"FAT IS A FEMINIST ISSUE..."

This astonishing and highly sensible book by a practicing psychotherapist tells you how to get off the diet/binge merry-go-round and lose weight by enjoying your food, your life, and yourself! Illustrated with actual case histories; complete with special sections on compulsive eating and *anorexia nervosa* (self-starvation).

A co-founder of the Women's Therapy Center Institute in New York and the Women's Therapy Center in London, Susie Orbach is a specialist in the treatment of compulsive eating.

Books by Susie Orbach

FAT IS A FEMINIST ISSUE
FAT IS A FEMINIST ISSUE II
HUNGER STRIKE:
The Anorectic's Struggle as a Metaphor for Our Age

with Luise Eichenbaum

UNDERSTANDING WOMEN:
A Feminist Psychoanalytic Approach
WHAT DO WOMEN WANT?
Exploding the Myth of Women's Dependency
BETWEEN WOMEN:
Love, Envy and Competition in Women's Friendships

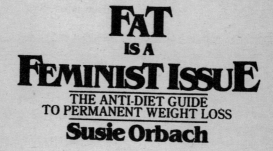

FAT IS A FEMINIST ISSUE

THE ANTI-DIET GUIDE
TO PERMANENT WEIGHT LOSS

Susie Orbach

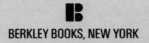

BERKLEY BOOKS, NEW YORK

FAT IS A FEMINIST ISSUE

A Berkley Book / published by arrangement with
the author

PRINTING HISTORY
Paddington Press edition published 1978
Berkley edition / April 1979
Berkley edition with new introduction / September 1990

ISBN: 0-425-09920-2

A BERKLEY BOOK ® TM 757,375
Berkley Books are published by The Berkley Publishing Group,
200 Madison Avenue, New York, New York 10016.
The name "BERKLEY" and the "B" logo
are trademarks belonging to Berkley Publishing Corporation.

PRINTED IN THE UNITED STATES OF AMERICA

10 9 8 7 6 5 4 3 2 1

For
Eleanor Anguti,
Carol Bloom
and
Lela Zaphiropoulos

Contents

Acknowledgments

Thanks are due to many, many people. First to Carol Munter, the original compulsive-eating and self-image group, and all the women with whom I have worked and who have shared their feelings about their bodies with me. Without these people there would be no book and nothing to say. Thanks too to all those people who have generously encouraged, helped and supported me in this work in one way or another over the past six years. They include Dale Bernstein, Patrick Byrne, Warren Cohen, Anne Cooke, Clare Dennis, Luise Eichenbaum, Peggy Eliot, Ian Franklin, Barbara Goldberg, Clara Caleo Green, Rose Heatley, Altheia Jones Lecointe, Eddie Lebar, Bob Lefferts, David McLanahan, Laurence Orbach, Ruth Orbach, Rosie Parker, Jeremy Pikser, Cathy Porter, Ron Radosh, Olly Rosengart, Julie Saj, Steve Sandler, David Skinner, DeeDee Skinner, Laura Schwartz, Michael Schwartz, Ann Snitow, Jimmy Traub, Redesign, Spare Rib and the Women's Therapy Centre.

Finally, four people have come through with

ix

support in immeasurable ways. Sara Baerwald has provided consistent no-nonsense support from afar. Malinda Coleman miraculously dropped everything to provide crucial help at a critical time. Gillian Slovo cared for me very well in the final stages. Joseph Schwartz came through in unimaginable ways providing love, support, patience, criticism, handholding and chicken soup throughout—my love and deep appreciation cannot express how important this has been to me.

All the case histories in this book are true. The names and places have been changed to protect the privacy of individuals and their families.

Preface

In March 1970, I went to the Alternate U on Sixth Avenue and 14th Street in New York City to register for a course on compulsive eating and self-image—women only. I walked into a room jammed with forty women of various sizes talking about their bodies and their eating habits. Carol Munter, the course organizer, visibly delighted by the turnout, was suggesting that we break up into four groups. It was the first time since the beginning of the women's liberation movement that women had dared to come forward for discussion groups specifically dealing with body image. The call for the course had seemed to me almost like a travesty—feminists concerned about how they looked! At the time we were used to rejecting male ideals of how we should look as projected in advertisements and movies. We were ostensibly happy in our blue jeans and work shirts. We were not used to discussing clothes or body size with our female friends; there was, in fact, a widespread feeling of relief that we could relax in our clothes and bodies and not worry about what was especially fashionable, provocative or appealing. We wore the clothes of rebellion and did not care what others thought. Or did we?

Before we divided into groups, Carol Munter mentioned two things. The first was that she knew someone who had lost a lot of weight without dieting; the second, that she had constructed in the closet next door a four-way mirror by pasting long strips of aluminum foil on the walls. Anyone who wanted could go into the closet and look at herself in private from all four sides for as long as she wanted. Carol thought these two things—non-dieting and self-acceptance—might be keys to weight loss. I scarcely paid attention. I was thinking, "What am I doing here? I often look at myself in the mirror, I'm not frightened to do that.... I'm slimmer than some, will the other women accept me?"

Our group set a meeting time for the following week and we all dispersed. I was confused, having anticipated a discussion of nutritional standards in the United States and the Third World, or perhaps a look at the food and fashion industries or the incidence of obesity in "rich countries." I was hesitant to explore the topic of compulsive eating outside the context of a political vocabulary—a vocabulary that looked at the relationship between patriarchy and Western society with the family as the lynch pin. I was uneasy but held on to the slogan that the personal is political.

I would not have gone back but for one thing. Despite my discomfort and need to compare myself with the other women, I also experienced an overwhelming relief to be in a group with women, fat and thin, who were all compulsive eaters. The problem had been named and perhaps I did not have to feel quite so ashamed. In the last year or so I had become quite used to talking about very personal topics in consciousness-raising groups and I was suddenly quite excited that Carol was suggesting we discuss in the same way a subject that had been so hidden and so private.

Six months later I left the group. I no longer defined myself as a compulsive eater and I had stabilized at a weight I found acceptable. It turned out to be rather higher than my previous Twiggy-like fantasies. Food no longer terrified me and I could live in my body. I find this knowledge continues to amaze me, so painful were those ten years of dieting, bingeing and self-hatred. So what had happened in the group that had produced this transformation? Really a lot!

We had taken the formula of a women's group and one by one we shared how we felt about our bodies, being attractive, food, eating, thinness, fatness and clothes. We detailed our previous diet histories and traded horror stories of doctors, psychiatrists, diet organizations, health farms and fasting. We knew enough to know that all our previous attempts at getting our bodes the right weight and shape had not worked. We wondered *why* we had wanted them so right, *what* was so powerful about looking a particular way that we had all tried and succeeded in losing weight dozens of times. We did not understand why we could not keep "it" off; why every time we neared the goal "it" would creep up, or why we always broke our diets. Why were we so plagued by our body size and shape?

We began asking new questions and coming up with new answers. We were a self-help group at the time when energy from the women's liberation movement sparked us all into rethinking many previously held assumptions. The creativity of the movement prepared a fertile soil in which feminist ideas, nurtured and developed in countless consciousness-raising groups, in mass marches and demonstrations, in organized political campaigns, found new applications and usefulness. Compulsive eating was one such area.

Compulsive eating is a very painful and, on the surface, self-destructive, activity. But feminism has taught us to be wary of this label. Feminism has taught us that activities that appear to be self-destructive are invariably adaptations, attempts to cope with the world. In our group, we turned our strongly held ideas about dieting and thinness upside down. Carol reminded us of her friend who lost weight without dieting. Slowly and unsurely we stopped dieting. Nothing terrible happened. My world did not collapse. Carol raised the central question; maybe we did not want to be thin. I dismissed that out of hand. Of course I wanted to be thin, I would be. . . . The dots turned out to hold the answer. Who I would be thin was different from who *I* was. I decided I did not want to be thin, there was not much in it. You were more hassled by men, you became a sex object. No, I definitely did not want to be thin.... I developed a new political reason for not being thin—I was not going to be like the fashion magazines wanted me to be; I was a Jewish beatnik and I would be *zaftig*. I relaxed, ate what I wanted, and wore clothes that were expressive of me. I even felt a little smug. I ignored the diet sheets in the newspapers, I enjoyed the different food phases I was going through and I walked down the street feeling increasingly confident. But the dots nagged. Why was I afraid of being thin? The things I was frightened of came into vision. I confronted them, always asking myself— how would it help to be fat in this situation? *What* would be more troublesome if I were thin? As the image of my fat and thin personality conflated, I began to lose weight. I felt a deep satisfaction that I could be a size that felt good for me and no longer obsessed with food. I promised myself I would not be responsible for depriving myself of the food I liked. I had learned a crucial lesson—that I could be the same person thin as I was fat. Satisfied, I left the group. Together we had developed a theory and practice that made sense. Carol and I went on to help other women sort through this problem. We ran groups. We became therapists and worked with women individually and together for five years.

This book is an attempt to share this work. It is my view of what we learned in that first group and then with the subsequent groups and individual women who shared their compulsive-eating problems with us. As such, this book is necessarily limited; it does not have enough scope to provide a comprehensive picture of compulsive eating, but it does address dimensions that have been missed by other people who work in the field. The observations and insights are drawn from women from the United States, Canada and England. They are all white and range in age from seventeen to sixty-five. They include grandmothers and single women. The women are from working-class backgrounds and middle- and upper-middle-income groups. I very much hope that this book will be useful to a wider audience, particularly black and Latin women, but I recognize that their cultural experience is different from those of the women with whom these ideas were developed and may therefore not address significant themes for them.

Compulsive eating has been studied by many different people, including psychiatrists, psychoanalysts, psychologists, doctors, nutritionists and endocrinologists.[1] By and large, the approach has been either to try to remove the resultant obesity or to treat the underlying cause of distress that has produced compulsive eating. Compulsive eating has never been strictly defined but what it has meant for me and the women I have worked with is:

Eating when you are not physically hungry.

Feeling out of control around food, submerged by either dieting or gorging.

Spending a good deal of time thinking and worrying about foot and fatness.

Scouring the latest diet for vital information.

Feeling awful about yourself as someone who is out of control.

Feeling awful about your body.

Our approach has been to see compulsive eating as *both* a symptom and a problem in itself. It is a symptom in the sense that the compulsive eater does not know how to cope with whatever underlies this behavior and turns to food. On the other hand, the compulsive-eating syndrome is so highly developed and painfully absorbing that it has to be addressed directly as the problem too. Consequently, we address both aspects. We explore and demystify the symptom to find out what is being expressed in the desire to be fat, in the fear of thinness and in the wish to fill and starve ourselves. At the same time we attempt to intervene directly so that the feelings and behavior around food can change. Underlying problems need to be exposed and separated, though not necessarily worked through. The perspective is always to see the social dimensions that have led women to choose compulsive eating as an adaptation to sexist pressure in contemporary society.

We are aware that contemporary preoccupation with thinness is both new and restricted to those Western nations that appear not to have food shortages. The food production in these countries is largely in the hands of multinational corporations.[2] They cover all aspects of the market from "high protein," "vitamin rich" foods and "wholesome, natural" foods, or dietetic candies, jellies, ice creams, milks and sodas. Women, as the most important purchasers of foods, are presented with a seemingly vast choice. They must choose wisely for their families' health and welfare. At the same time every woman is continually confronted with images of slimness and trimness and advice on how to eat sensibly, lose weight and have a happy life. This general concern with thinness affects both women and men, and people are often driven to reduce their size when they were not previously over large. Thus starts a cycle of food deprivation and compulsive eating. Women are especially susceptible to these demands to lose weight because they are brought up to conform to an image of womanhood that places importance on body size and shape. We are taught that we must both blend in and stand out—a contradictory message indeed.

Men are increasingly being affected by similar pressures and although I have worked with several men, I have not attempted to formulate a theory that describes how sexism affects men's body size.

This book is written as a self-help manual. However, therapists may wish to incorporate this method into their own work with compulsive eaters.[3]

To all women who suffer from the problem of compulsive eating, I hope that the accumulated experience of other women as expressed in this book will speak to you.

Susie Orbach
London, 1978

Introduction to new edition

It is no more than thirteen years since I sat down to write FIFI *(FAT IS A FEMINIST ISSUE ...)*. As a woman who had found personal relief from my compulsive eating, and as a psychotherapist who had worked with numerous groups and individual women (and some men) who had eating problems, I wanted to share what I had learned with a wider audience. My hope was that FIFI could encourage those women preoccupied with body-image difficulties to think through their eating problems and their relationship to their bodies with a new perspective. I hoped that psychotherapists might incorporate the methods outlined in FIFI into their clinical practices, so that they might hear with a different ear the anguish and distress hidden behind their patients' and clients' reports of their latest diet or binge episode.

Much to my surprise, the book struck a powerful chord in hundreds of thousands of women. Compulsive eating and its sister conditions – bulimia and anorexia – came out of the closet. Hundreds of self-help groups started up; Spare Tyre Theatre Company formed, to write and produce musical plays on the topic; numerous TV documentaries and several films were made; approaches were made to manufacturers of women's clothing to make attractive styles in all sizes; *Cosmopolitan* dropped its diet column; many women were able to give up dieting and accept their bodies at sizes that had repulsed them before. I began to feel that women were fighting back and contesting the blanket message that they should be thin. I was optimistic that the children being raised now might be free of these disabling body-image and eating problems that had so beset my generation.

Thirteen years on, we discover the dismaying fact that 80 per cent of San Franciscan girls are dieting because even the scrawny ones believe that they are "overweight". Girls from the age of nine right through to women in their sixties have absorbed the message that they can solve emotional problems, sexual problems, family problems, relationship problems, work problems – all through the transformation of their body size. Obsession and preoccupation with the body has *increased* rather than abated. We live in a culture that continues to be obsessed with women's body size and body shape – that sees fatness and thinness as ultimate statements about people's worth rather than descriptions of the ratio of fat body tissue and lean body tissue.

The current aesthetic of thinness forces cruel pressures on the individual women. Few women are naturally thin, or indeed naturally any size. We are a variety of sizes. But the thin aesthethic which has dominated the last twenty years has put women in the impossible position of feeling that they must curb their appetites and their food intake. They must do this at the same time that they feed others and express their caring and concern for them through the food they prepare and serve. In other words, women absorb a powerfully contradictory message vis a vis food and eating. It is good for others, but bad for the woman herself; healthy for others, harmful to the woman herself; full of love and nurturance for others, full of self-indulgence to herself.

Much as I would rather it were not so, the problems raised in FIFI are still with us. Some issues have changed, but many of those I hoped to raise thirteen years ago are even more pressing now. The conditions that have given rise to women's eating problems have only begun to shift. Some of the changes are amusing. In the 1970s, nutritional theory elevated cheese and dairy products as good wholesome foods. Pasta and potatoes were heavily caloric and necessarily bad. Today's nutritional theory tells us that cheese and dairy products are full of animal fat and bad, while pasta and potatoes are carbohydrates – the "in" food category! As women scurry to find information outside themselves about what and how they should be eating, they are buffeted by ever-changing nutritional theories purporting to be the truth.

Other changes are more sinister. Models today are younger and younger, their bodies resembling not so much those of women as those of the pre-adolescents and adolescents that they are. The weight of those winning beauty contests has gone down, and despite the fact that it is estimated that 50% of North American women weigh well above the "recommended" numbers on the height/weight tables, slimness has not declined as an aesthetic; rather it has captured the desire of more and more people and come to represent the longings of more and more women. Women are still all too often seen as sexual objects for others. Whether at home or at work, their self-esteem can

still depend in large measure on how they feel about
their bodies. Along with the escalation of slimness
and its reach into ever-younger sections of the population, there is a demand that we should be fitter. The
emphasis on health and the exercise club has given
women access to sports and their physicality in a new
way. At the same time, however, they are now subject
to a new pressure: the designer body.

Over the last decade, many individual women have
been able to make much-wanted changes in their personal lives. However, in the public sphere feminine
values find little place and evidence of women's political and social power is still limited. In exchange for
our desire to transform our lives, we are given back
the body and the correct feeding of others and ourselves as the arena in which we should concentrate.
We are in a transitional period, and the link between
our old identities and roles and our new ones is something we know only too well about – preoccupation
with the body and a concern about the food we eat.

As women attempt to deal with their new (barely
allowed) aspirations and cope with their old expectations of self, the categories of fat and thin are offered
as solutions to complex problems. The new career
woman is always thin. The competent mother is always thin. The middle-aged woman returning to work
is always thin. Images of the new women are always
presented to us as *thin,* and such ideas about thinness
become insinuated into each woman's sense of herself
so that she sees thinness as an important part of the
way she should be.

In FIFI I have talked about fat, thin, and overweight
as they are used by the women I have worked with.
This means that they are not so much descriptions of
body size as they are emotional categories: emotional

categories that carry the weight of cultural dictates we have all internalized. Re-reading the text, I think it would be helpful if quote marks could surround the words "fat", "thin" and "overweight". In this way we might be able to recognize the extent to which these words are so much more physically descriptive. They carry social meaning, fantasies, projections and mis-perceptions. When I write about what a woman's "fat" might mean or might be saying about her, I am not writing about fat *per se,* but about her fantasies. Indeed, the woman may not be large or fat at all. It may be her imagination – aided by a culture obsessed with making a fetish of the female form – that has al-lowed her to construe that her body is fat. She may be fat; she may be well within what anyone might con-sider the norm; she may even be very skinny and still use the word "fat" to convey how she feels about her body. So when I speak of "fat" or "thin" or "over-weight", I am talking about *a state of mind.* I am ex-ploring what seeing herself in this way means for her. I am writing about the need to decode the food and body-image metaphors that have become a woman's language. To be sure, these are not always easy to un-derstand. We need to understand what a woman is saying when she uses her body to express difficult emotional issues. We need to understand why it is safer to say, "I need to go on a diet" than "I feel hurt or upset or in conflict."

We don't tell one another that we are in screaming anguish; we tell one another we feel bad that we are fat. We don't tell one another about our desperation and feelings of impotence; we say that if we were thin, things would be so much better. We don't tell one an-other we feel invisible and unrecognized; we become anorexic and force that recognition on others.

Because food and the body has become an arena in which women have been allowed to express themselves, food and the body become a language they communicate with. We may not be able to decipher the code at first glance, but if we look and listen and ask, we develop the capacity to comprehend the messages that are encoded in women's relationship to food. As we decode them, we see how intimately linked they are to the psychological conditions created by our present social climate.

Today, a decade and a half of feminism have allowed women to honour their experiences, to investigate these for themselves and analyze what they have meant. We have legitimated the body as a proper area for political concern. As we have done so, we have begun to understand the complex messages each of us attempts to express through our body and our eating. We discover that we have been trying to come to terms with what the culture at large represents for us as femininity, and how we wish to represent ourselves. We discover how impossible that is, and our own ideas about ourselves are inextricable from everything we have grown up with. We discover how much our eating and non-eating behaviors are attempts to stifle inner conflicts we feel; how our preoccupations with the body are manifestations of our desire to work things out in the arena we have been given. We translate life problems into food problems or body problems. We imagine that we can fix what is wrong in the world – the large world or our own smaller personal worlds – by eating/not eating/getting bigger/getting smaller. We refuse to accept our powerlessness and so we manipulate ourselves fantasizing that we can have power through self-transformation.

We discover how we deal with indigestible facts and

feelings by eating them; how we seek soothing and solace for hurt in eating or in not eating; how we gather self-esteem through what we do or do not put in our bodies. There is an intricate interplay between our bodies and what we allow them to have, and our unconscious and conscious beliefs about our entitlements. For women today, their relationship to food is generally so fraught and problematic that each eating episode tells a story – a story of inner pain and anguish, of hope, of self-disgust, of the attempt to care for self. As we patiently decode these messages and their contradictory aspects, we learn much about women's desires and the restraints they have internalized. We also learn much about our need for soothing and the brutality with which we try to squash our needs.

It is time once again to question our culture's preoccupation with women's body image. We need to challenge the idea that women should be a particular size and shape, and that happiness or contentment is contingent on attaining it. We need to resist the huge advertising campaigns – profitable to the companies concerned, but harmful to women – that exhort us to dress/eat/feed others and ourselves in specific ways. It is equally important to understand the particular meanings that "fat" and "thin" have come to have for women today, and to help women overcome their eating problems and live with ease in their bodies.

At the same time, we need to question our social practices so that the next generation of girls and women will not suffer from such disabling and distressing feelings about their bodies and their food.

Susie Orbach
London, 1990

FAT IS A FEMINIST ISSUE

Introduction

Obesity and overeating have joined sex as central issues in the lives of many women today. In the United States, 50 percent of women are estimated to be overweight. Every women's magazine has a diet column. Diet doctors and clinics flourish. The names of diet foods are now part of our general vocabulary. Physical fitness and beauty are every woman's goals. While this preoccupation with fat and food has become so common that we tend to take it for granted, being fat, feeling fat and the compulsion to overeat are, in fact, serious and painful experiences for the women involved.

3

Being fat isolates and invalidates a woman. Almost inevitably, the explanations offered for fatness point a finger at the failure of women themselves to control their weight, control their appetites and control their impulses. Women suffering from the problem of compulsive eating endure a double anguish: feeling out of step with the rest of society, and believing that it is all their own fault.

The number of women who have problems with weight and compulsive eating is large and growing. Owing to the emotional distress involved and the fact that the many varied solutions offered to women in the past have not worked, a new psychotherapy to deal with compulsive eating has had to evolve within the context of the movement for women's liberation. This new psychotherapy represents a feminist rethinking of traditional psychoanalysis.

A psychoanalytic approach has much to offer toward a solution to compulsive-eating problems. It provides ways for exploring the roots of such problems in early experiences. It shows us how we develop our adult personalities, most importantly our sexual identity—how a female baby becomes a girl and then a woman, and how a male baby becomes a boy and then a man. Psychoanalytic insight helps us to understand what getting fat and overeating mean to individual women—by explaining their conscious or unconscious acts.

An approach based exclusively on classical psychoanalysis, without a feminist perspective is, however, inadequate. Since the Second World War, psychiatry has, by and large, told unhappy women that their discontent represents an inability to

resolve the "Oedipal constellation." Female fatness
has been diagnosed as an obsessive-compulsive
symptom related to separation-individuation, nar-
cissism and insufficient ego development.[1] Being
overweight is seen as a deviance and anti-men.
Overeating and obesity have been reduced to
character defects, rather than perceived as the
expression of painful and conflicting experiences.
Furthermore, rather than attempting to uncover
and confront women's bad feelings about their
bodies or toward food, professionals concerned
themselves with the problem of how to get the
women thin. So, after the psychiatrists, analysts and
clinical psychologists proved unsuccessful, experimental workers looked for biological and even
genetic reasons for obesity. None of these approaches has had convincing, lasting results. None
of them has addressed the central issues of
compulsive eating which are rooted in the social
inequality of women.

A feminist perspective to the problem of
women's compulsive eating is essential if we are to
move on from the ineffective blame-the-victim
approach[2] and the unsatisfactory adjustment model
of treatment. While psychoanalysis gives us useful
tools to discover the deepest sources of emotional
distress, feminism insists that those painful personal
experiences derive from the social context into
which female babies are born, and within which
they develop to become adult women. The fact that
compulsive eating is overwhelmingly a woman's
problem suggests that it has something to do with
the experience of being female in our society.
Feminism argues that being fat represents an
attempt to break free of society's sex stereotypes.

Getting fat can thus be understood as a definite and purposeful act; it is a directed, conscious or unconscious, challenge to sex-role stereotyping and culturally defined experience of womanhood.

Fat is a social disease, and fat is a feminist issue. Fat is *not* about lack of self-control or lack of will power. Fat *is* about protection, sex, nurturance, strength, boundaries, mothering, substance, assertion and rage. It is a response to the inequality of the sexes. Fat expresses experiences of women today in ways that are seldom examined and even more seldom treated. While becoming fat does not alter the roots of sexual oppression, an examination of the underlying causes or unconscious motivation that lead women to compulsive eating suggests new treatment possibilities. Unlike most weight-reducing schemes, our new therapeutic approach does not reinforce the oppressive social roles that lead women into compulsive eating in the first place. What is it about the social position of women that leads them to respond to it by getting fat?

The current ideological justification for inequality of the sexes has been built on the concept of the innate differences between women and men. Women alone can give birth to and breast-feed their infants and, as a result, a primary dependency relationship develops between mother and child. While this biological capacity is the only known genetic difference between men and women,[3] it is used as the basis on which to divide unequally women and men's labor, power, roles and expectations. The division of labor has become institutionalized. Woman's capacity to reproduce and provide nourishment has relegated her to the care and socialization of children.

The relegation of women to the social roles of wife and mother has several significant consequences that contribute to the problem of fat. First, in order to become a wife and mother, a woman has to have a man. Getting a man is presented as an almost unattainable and yet essential goal. To get a man, a woman has to learn to regard herself as an item, a commodity, a sex object. Much of her experience and identity depends on how she and others see her. As John Berger says in *Ways of Seeing*:

Men *act* and women *appear*. Men look at women. Women watch themselves being looked at. This determines not only most relations between men and women, but also the relation of women to themselves.[4]

This emphasis on presentation as the central aspect of a woman's existence makes her extremely self-conscious. It demands that she occupy herself with a self-image that others will find pleasing and attractive—an image that will immediately convey what kind of woman she is. She must observe and evaluate herself, scrutinizing every detail of herself as though she were an outside judge. She attempts to make herself in the image of womanhood presented by billboards, newspapers, magazines and television. The media present women either in a sexual context or within the family, reflecting a woman's two prescribed roles, first as a sex object, and then as a mother. She is brought up to marry by "catching" a man with her good looks and pleasing manner. To do this she must look appealing, earthy, sensual, sexual, virginal, innocent, reliable, daring, mysterious, coquettish and thin. In other words, she offers her self-image on the marriage marketplace. As a married woman, her sexuality will be sanctioned and her economic needs will be looked after. She will have achieved the first step of womanhood.

Since women are taught to see themselves from the outside as candidates for men, they become prey to the huge fashion and diet industries that first set up the ideal images and then exhort women to meet them. The message is loud and clear—the woman's body is not her own. The woman's body is not satisfactory as it is. It must be thin, free of "unwanted hair," deodorized, perfumed and clothed. It must conform to an ideal physical type. Family and school socialization teaches girls to groom themselves properly. Furthermore, the job is never-ending, for the image changes from year to year. In the early 1960s, the only way to feel acceptable was to be skinny and flat chested with long straight hair. The first of these was achieved by near starvation, the second, by binding one's breasts with an ace bandage and the third, by ironing one's hair. Then in the early 1970s, the look was curly hair and full breasts. Just as styles in clothes change seasonally, so women's bodies are expected to change to fit these fashions. Long and skinny one year, petite and demure the next, women are continually manipulated by images of proper womanhood, which are extremely powerful because they are presented as the only reality. To ignore them means to risk being an outcast. Women are urged to conform, to help out the economy by continuous consumption of goods and clothing that are quickly made unwearable by the next season's fashion styles in clothes and body shapes. In the background, a ten billion dollar industry waits to remold bodies to the latest fashion. In this way, women are caught in an attempt to conform to a standard that is *externally* defined and constantly changing. But these models of femininity are experienced by women as unreal, frightening and unattainable. They produce a picture that is far removed from the reality of women's day-to-day lives.

The one constant in these images is that a woman must be thin. For many women, compulsive eating and being fat have become one way to avoid being marketed or seen as the ideal woman: "My fat says 'screw you' to all who want me to be the perfect mom, sweetheart, maid and whore. Take me for who *I* am, not for who I'm supposed to be. If you are really interested in *me*, you can wade through the layers and find out who I am." In this way, fat expresses a rebellion against the powerlessness of the woman, against the pressure to look and act in a certain way and against being evaluated on her ability to create an image of herself.

Becoming fat is, thus, a woman's response to the first step in the process of fulfilling a prescribed social role which requires her to shape herself to an externally imposed image in order to catch a man. But a second stage in this process takes place after she achieves that goal, after she has become a wife and mother.

For a mother, everyone else's needs come first. Mothers are the unpaid managers of small, essential, complex and demanding organizations. They may not control the financial arrangements of this minicorporation or the major decisions on location or capital expenditure, but they do generally control the day-to-day operations. For her keep, the mother works an estimated ten hours a day (eighteen, if she has a second job outside the home) making sure that the food is purchased and prepared, the children's clothes, toys and books are in place, and that the father's effects are at the ready. She makes the house habitable, clean and comfy; she does the social secretarial work of arranging for the family to spend time with relatives and friends; she provides a baby-sitting and chauffeur-escort service for her children. As babies and children, we are all cared for. As adults, however, women are expected to feed and clean not only their babies but also their husbands, and only then, themselves.

In this role women experience particular pressure over food and eating. After the birth of each baby, breasts or bottle becomes a major issue. The mother is often made to feel insecure about her adequacy to perform her fundamental job. In the hospital the baby is weighed after each feed to see if the mother's breasts have enough milk. Pediatricians and baby-care books bombard the new mother with authoritative but conflicting advice about, for example, scheduled versus demand feeding, composition of the formula or the introduction of solid foods. As her children grow older, a woman continues to be reminded that her feeding skills are inadequate. To the tune of billions of dollars a year, the food industry counsels her on how, when and what she should feed her charges. The advertisements cajole her into providing nutritious breakfasts, munchy snacks, and wholesome dinners. Media preoccupation with good housekeeping and, particularly, with good food and good feeding, serves as a yardstick by which to measure the mother's ever-failing performance. This preoccupation colonizes food preparation so that the housewife is presented with a list of "do's" and "don'ts" so contradictory that it is a wonder that anything gets produced in the kitchen at all. It is not surprising that a woman quickly learns not to trust her own impulses, either in feeding her family or in listening to her own needs when she feeds herself.

During the period in her life which is devoted to child rearing, the woman is constantly making sure that others' lives run smoothly. She does this without thinking seriously that she is working at a full-time job. Her own experience of everyday life is as midwife to others' activities. While she is preparing her children to become future workers, and enabling her husband to be a more "effective" producer, her role is to produce and reproduce workers. In this capacity she is constantly giving out without receiving the credit that would validate her social worth.

In a capitalist society everyone is defined by their job. A higher status is given to businessmen, academics and professionals than to production and service workers. Women's work in the home falls into the service and production category. Although often described as menial, deemed creative, dismissed as easy, or revered as god-given, women's work is seen as existing outside the production process and therefore devalued. Women as a group are allowed less expression than the men in their social class. However oppressed men are by a class society, they hold more power than women. Every man has to watch out for his boss. Every woman has to watch out lest her man not approve. The standards and views of the day are male. Women are seen as different from normal people

(who are men), they are seen as "other."⁵ They are
not accepted as equal human beings with men. Their
full identity is not supported by the society in which
they grow up. This leads to confusion for women.
Women are trapped in the role of an alien, yet
delegated responsibility for making sure that others'
lives are productive.

Since women are not accepted as equal human
beings but are nevertheless expected to devote
enormous energy to the lives of others, the
distinctions between their own lives and the lives of
those close to them may become blurred. Merging
with others, feeding others, not knowing how to
make space for themselves are frequent themes for
women. Mothers are constantly giving out and
feeding the world; everyone else's needs are
primary. That they feel confusion about their own
bodily needs is not surprising and there may be few
ways of noting their personal concerns. A form of
giving to and replenishing oneself is through food.
"I eat a lot because I'm always stoking myself up for
the days's encounters. I look after my family, my
mother and any number of people who pass in and
out of my day. I feel empty with all this giving so I
eat to fill up the spaces and give me sustenance to go
on giving to the world." The resulting fat has the
function of making the space for which women
crave. It is an attempt to answer the question, "If I
am constantly giving myself to everyone, where do I
begin and end?" We want to look and be substantial.
We want to be bigger than society will let us. We
want to take up as much space as the other sex. "If I
get bigger like a man then maybe I'll get taken
seriously as is a man."

What happens to the woman who does not fit the

social role? Although the image of ideal sexual object and all-competent mother is socially pervasive, it is not only limiting and unattainable, but it also fails to correspond to the reality of many, many women's lives today. Most women today do still marry and have children. But many also continue to work outside the home after marriage, either to meet economic needs or in an attempt to break the limits of their social role. Women continually juggle with the many different aspects of their personalities which are developed and expressed at great cost against this unfriendly background. In this context, just as many women first become fat in an attempt to avoid being made into sexual objects at the beginning of their adult lives, so many women remain fat as a way of neutralizing their sexual identity in the eyes of others who are important to them as their life progresses. In this way, they can hope to be taken seriously in their working lives outside the home. It is unusual for women to be accepted for their competence in this sphere. When they lose weight, that is, begin to look like a perfect female, they find themselves being treated frivolously by their male colleagues. When women are thin, they *are* treated frivolously: thin-sexy-incompetent worker. But if a woman loses weight, she herself may not yet be able to separate thinness from the packaged sexuality around her which simultaneously defines her as incompetent. It is difficult to conform to one image that society would have you fit (thin) without also being the other image (sexy female). "When I'm fat, I feel I can hold my own. Whenever I get thin I feel I'm being treated like a little doll who doesn't know which end is up."

We have seen how fat is a symbolic rejection of

the limitations of women's role, an adaptation that many women use in the burdensome attempt to pursue their individual lives within the proscriptions of their social function. But in order to understand more about the way that overweight and, in particular, overeating, function in the lives of individual women, we must examine the process by which they are initially taught their social role. It is a complex and ironic process, for women are prepared for this life of inequality by other women who themselves suffer its limitations—their mothers. The feminist perspective reveals that compulsive eating is, in fact, an expression of the complex relationships between mothers and daughters.

If a woman's social role is to become a mother, nurturing—feeding the family in the widest possible sense—is the mother's central job. By and large, it is only within the family that a woman has any social power. Her competence as a mother and her ability to be an emotional support for her family defines her and provides her with a recognized context within which to exist. For a mother, a crucial part of the maternal role is to help her daughter, as her mother did before her, to make a smooth transition into the female social role. From her mother, the young girl learns who she herself is and can be. The mother provides her with a model of feminine behavior, and directs the daughter's behavior in particular ways.

But the world the mother must present to her daughter is one of unequal relationships, between parent and child, authority and powerlessness, man and woman. The child is exposed to the world of power relationships by a unit that itself produces and reproduces perhaps the most fundamental of these inequalities. Within the family, an inferior sense of self is instilled into little girls.[6] While it is obvious that the growing-up process for girls and boys is vastly different, what may be less apparent is that to prepare her daughter for a life of inequality, the mother tries to hold back her child's desires to be a powerful, autonomous, self-directed, energetic and productive human being. From an early age, the young girl is encouraged to accept this rupture in her development and is guided to cope with this loss by putting her energy into taking care of others. Her own needs for emotional support and growth will be satisfied if she can convert them into giving to others.

Meanwhile, little boys are taught to accept emotional support without learning how to give this kind of nurturing and loving in return. Therefore, when a young woman finally achieves the social reward of marriage, she finds that it rarely provides either the nurture she still needs, or an opportunity for independence and self-development. To be a woman is to live with the tension of giving and not getting; and the mother and daughter involved in the process leading to this conclusion are inevitably bound up in ambivalence, difficulty and conflict.

If we look at it from the mother's point of view, the process of leading her daughter to adult womanhood is ambivalent for several reasons. The first is the question of independence. The mother, who has been prepared for a life of giving, finds her feeding, nurturing and child-rearing capacity—so integral to her success in her social role—satisfied. She needs to be needed and has indeed fulfilled herself as a "good mother" by attentively feeding her child. Thus, mothers do and do not want their daughters to leave them. They do because the maternal role also requires them to prepare their daughters for eventual independence: to fail at this is to fail at motherhood. On the other hand, to succeed at this signals the end of motherhood. We have seen that of the limited roles that have been available to women in this century, motherhood is the only one in which women have legitimate power. Therefore, their personal success at being mothers results in their loss of power. Their personal success is a dead end; it does not lead on to the creation of a new, equally powerful role.

The mother's ambivalence is, however, even more painful in that mothers do and do not want their daughters to be like them. For a daughter to be like her mother is a way, at least partially, to validate the mother's life. But, the mother's life remains an invalidated life and the daughter's act of reproducing her mother's lifestyle can be no more than a perpetuation of powerlessness. In her love for her daughter, the mother must inevitably want a different life for her.

Nevertheless, mothers may feel ambivalent about the changing opportunities available to their daughters which were not available to them. They may be jealous of these opportunities, and fearful of their daughters' welfare in a world they know to be hostile to women, at the same time as they acquire some indirect satisfaction at their daughters' ambition and success. While a mother must be a mother, a daughter can be ambitious and engaged in the world.

Let us now look at these conflicts from the daughter's point of view. Daughters do and do not want to leave their mothers. For a daughter to leave is for her to become independent, part of the world, to signal her emergence as a female adult. However, this autonomy itself causes problems. As we have seen, independence in the world is not yet an option for female adults. Daughters feel ambivalent about their opportunities in the world; they are ill-prepared to take them up, as they have learned both from the culture at large and from their own mothers.

Daughters identify with the powerlessness of their mothers as women in a patriarchal society. They have been brought up to be like their mothers. But daughters both do and do not want to be like their mothers. While they identify with their mothers as women, as givers, as caretakers, they may nevertheless desire a different experience of womanhood. In leaving, in moving outside the prescribed female role, the daughter may feel she is betraying her mother or is showing her up by doing "better." She may also feel nervous about being on shaky, untested ground. Furthermore, if a daughter identifies with her mother's powerlessness, she may see her role as that of taking care of her mother—to provide her mother with the love, care and interest she never received. She becomes her mother's mother? Leaving becomes even more of a betrayal.

How do these ambivalences and conflicts in the mother-daughter relationship come to express themselves in fat, food and feeding? How is each adult woman who suffers from compulsive eating expressing what happened to her with her mother. It is obvious that feeding plays a crucial part in the relationship of mother and child, whatever the child's sex. Within the whole spectrum of nurturing activities expected of mothers, physical feeding is the most fundamental—indeed, instinctive. A mother's breasts provide food for her children, virtually without any conscious act on her own part, whereas all other nurturing activities, including the vital provision of emotional support, must be learned.

Because of her ambivalence toward her daughter, a mother's willingness to provide her with sensitive nurturing, both physically and emotionally, can be undermined. Both female and male babies experience their first love relationships with the mother, but early on the mother must withhold a certain degree of support and sustenance from her daughter, in order to teach her the ways of womanhood. This has specific consequences. In *Little Girls,*[7] Elena Gianini Belotti cites a study of mothers' attitudes and actions when feeding their babies. In a sample of babies of both sexes, 99 percent of boys were breast-fed, while only 66 percent of girls were. Girls were weaned significantly earlier than boys and spent 50 percent less time feeding (in the case of breast- and bottle-feeds this meant much smaller feeds than the boys'). Thus, daughters are often fed less well, less attentively and less sensitively than they need. Inappropriate and insensitive physical feeding is subsequently paralleled unconsciously by inadequate emotional feeding.

While unconsciously the mother may not be nurturing her daughter well, she gives up feeding her daughter only reluctantly. In the absence of an alternative role, the distinction between herself and her child now outside the womb may become blurred. The mother may see her child as a product, a possession or an extension of herself. Thus, the mother has an interest in retaining control over how much, what, when and how her child eats. She needs to encourage this initial dependency for her own social survival.

There may be great ambivalence about feeding and nurturing. A mother must make sure her daughter is not overfed in case she becomes greedy and overweight—a terrible fate for a girl. She must make sure the child looks healthy—this is normally associated with a certain roundness—and she needs the child to depend on her; for who else is she, if she is not seen as mother? Yet she may also dislike this dependency, which ties her down, drains her and prevents her from directing her energies elsewhere. Finally, she must prepare her daughter to become the future nurturer and feeder of someone else—her daughter's future child, lover, husband or parents. She must teach her daughter to be concerned with feeding and nourishing others at the cost of not fully developing herself.

Meanwhile, on the daughter's side, as she develops from child to woman, the daughter's feeding of herself can become a symbolic response to both the physical and emotional deprivation she suffered as a child, an expression of her fraught intimacy with her mother. As the child gets more adept, she begins to feed herself and select her own foods, producing a developing sense of independence of the mother. But this break causes conflict for the daughter. On the one hand, the daughter wants to move away and learn to take care of herself; on the other hand, this ability to nurture herself suggests a rejection of the mother. This rejection takes on a deep significance because of the social limitation of the woman's role in patriarchal society. If the mother is not needed as mother, who will she be? The daughter feels guilty about destroying her mother's only role. As she seeks emotional sustenance through other social relationships, the adult daughter may continue to suffer deprivation, as her own partner has, very often, not learned to give. She turns to eating in the search for love, comfort, warmth and support—for that indefinable something that seems never to be there.

Compulsive eating becomes a way of expressing either side of this conflict. In overfeeding herself, the daughter may be trying to reject her mother's role while at the same time reproaching the mother for inadequate nurturing; or she may be attempting to retain a sense of identity with her mother. Popular culture abounds with evidence of the symbolic value that food and fat hold between mothers and daughters. In *Lady Oracle*,[8] for example, Margaret Atwood shows how the daughter's fat becomes a weapon in her battle with her mother. When her mother gives Joan a clothing allowance as an incentive to reduce, Joan deliberately buys clothes that flaunt her size and finally, with the purchase of a lime-green carcoat, succeeds in reducing her mother to tears:

> My mother had never cried where I could see her and I was dismayed, but elated too at this evidence of my power, my only power. I had defeated her; I wouldn't ever let her make me over in her image, thin and beautiful.

Similarly, in the movie, *Summer Wishes, Winter Dreams,* when the mother criticizes her daughter's size, the latter blasts back that her fat is her own, that it is something for which she alone is responsible, that it is something her mother cannot take away too.

Women engaged in exploring their compulsive eating in relation to their mothers have come to the following varied realizations:

My fat says to my mother: "I'm substantial. I can protect myself. I can go out into the world."

My fat says to my mother: "Look at me. I'm a mess; I don't know how to take care of myself. You can still be my mother."

My fat says to my mother: "I'm going out in the world. I can't take you with me but I can take a part of you that's connected to me. My body is from yours. My fat is connected to you. This way I can still have you with me."

My fat says to my mother: "I'm leaving you but I still need you. My fat lets you know I'm not really able to take care of myself."

For the compulsive eater, fat has much symbolic meaning which makes sense within a feminist context. Fat is a response to the many oppressive manifestations of a sexist culture. Fat is a way of saying "no" to powerlessness and self-denial, to a limiting sexual expression which demands that females look and act a certain way, and to an image of womanhood that defines a specific social role. Fat offends Western ideals of female beauty and, as such, every "overweight" woman creates a crack in the popular culture's ability to make us mere products. Fat also expresses the tension in the mother-daughter relationship, the relationship which has been allocated the feminization of the female. This relationship is bound to be difficult in a patriarchal society because it demands that the already oppressed mothers become the teachers, preparers and enforcers of the oppression that society will visit on their daughters.

While fat serves the symbolic function of rejecting the way by which society distorts women and their relationships with others, particularly in the critical relationship between mothers and daughters, getting fat remains an unhappy and unsatisfactory attempt to resolve these conflicts. It is a painful price to pay, whether a woman is trying to conform to society's expectations or attempting to forge a new identity.

When something is "amiss" in this way, we can expect a psychological imbalance and reaction. Few things could be more "amiss" than the attempt of a patriarchal culture to inhibit a young girl's desires to be creative and expressive, to push her almost exclusively into restrictive gender-linked activities, thoughts and feelings. A woman's psychological development is structured in such a way as to prepare her for a life of inequality, but this straitjacket is not accepted lightly and invariably causes a "reaction." Psychological disturbance often distorts a person's physiological capacity: ability to eat, sleep, talk or enjoy sexual activity. I suggest that one of the reasons we find so many women suffering from eating disorders is because the social relationship between feeder and fed, between mother and daughter, fraught as it is with ambivalence and hostility, becomes a suitable mechanism for distortion and rebellion.

An examination of the symbolic meanings of fat provides insight into individual woman's experience in patriarchal culture. Fat is an adaptation to the oppression of women and, as such, it may be an unsatisfying personal solution and an ineffectual political attack. It is to this problem that our compulsive-eating therapy speaks, and it is within a feminist context that this is developed in the following chapters.

What is fat about for the compulsive eater?

Many people who are compulsive eaters underestimate the connection between their eating and body size. The compulsive eater often experiences her eating as chaotic, out of control, self-destructive and an example of her lack of will power. At the same time, however, she may say that really she just likes to eat a lot and is too greedy for her own good and that if it were not for the pounds and inches all this eating put on, she would be quite content. Some women say that if only there was a magic pill that allowed them to eat and eat incessantly while remaining at their ideal size, they would be quite happy. Indeed, women have had bypass surgery to achieve this state. So it is clear that people do see a connection between overeating and obesity and they attempt, through various deprivation schemes, to keep their overeating to a minimum so that they are not too fat.

What is crucial about this connection from the point of view of breaking the cycle of compulsive eating/dieting, however, is something often overlooked or misunderstood, both by compulsive eaters themselves and by those who try to help them. This is the idea that compulsive eating is linked to a desire to get fat. Now this point is not very obvious and can be difficult to understand. However, it is vital that we address it when trying to understand the immovability of the compulsive eater's seemingly bizarre relationship with food.

If one recognizes that compulsive-eating habits express an interest in being large, many things fall into place and the possibility of breaking the addiction to food is there.

Compulsive eating is a very, very painful activity. Behind the self-deprecating jokes is a person who suffers enormously. Much of her life is centered on food, what she can and cannot eat, what she will or will not eat, what she has or has not eaten and when she will or will not eat next. Typically, she cannot leave one mouthful of food on her plate and finds herself eating both at mealtimes and all through the day, evening or night. Much of her eating is done in secret or with eating friends, while at public meals she is the professional dieter and much admired for her abstinence. If she wants to eat cake she will go to the bakery and pretend that the cheesecake she buys is for her daughter or a friend, she will have it wrapped and only dare to eat it out in the open when she thinks no one will spot her. Alternatively she will buy some candy and hide it in her pocket, stealthily putting it into her mouth while she walks or drives along the street. The obsession with food carries with it an enormous amount of self-disgust, loathing and shame. These feelings arise from the experience of being out of control around food and compulsive eaters try numerous ways to discipline themselves. Many think that if they do not have access to food they will be alright. Therefore, if a compulsive eater lives alone her kitchen closets and refrigerator will probably contain only the most meager range of foods. The kitchen will seem almost medicinal with its skim milk, ice milk, cottage cheese, dietetic sodas and jellies that masquerade as real food.

Alison, a twenty-nine-year-old zoologist, explained the pitfalls in her system of banning enjoyable foods from her apartment. She woke up in the middle of the night and felt driven to eat. She had been bingeing all evening so there was virtually nothing except dry cereal in the apartment left to eat. For the last two weeks she had had in mind a batch of homemade chocolate-chip cookies she had baked for Greg, her upstairs neighbor. Greg had gone away on vacation and Alison knew that there were still some cookies left because, while watering his plants, she noticed the cookie tin sitting on the kitchen counter. She got out of bed and took the keys to get into his apartment, found the cookies and stood there eating them all. She felt she could not just have one or two because that would not be enough, and if she ate a substantial number, when he returned, Greg would realize some were missing.

Alison's solution was to stand in his freezing cold apartment and eat the lot hoping that when he returned he would not remember that he had left any cookies at all.

If the compulsive eater lives with others, the kitchen is more likely to be full of appetizing foods that she denies herself or feels she must deny herself. Helen, a fifty-year-old mother of two who has been watching her weight for the last thirty years, is so petrified of the food in her house that she has arranged with her husband that he lock the kitchen door at night. She has a coffee percolator by her bed and celery and carrots on ice and she is banned from the kitchen on all occasions except when preparing family meals and eating her dietetic version of them. Her situation is just an extreme example of what many compulsive eaters go through in their attempts to stay away from food.

Helen brought her husband in on her problem but for Alison it was of paramount importance that nobody else knew that she was eating in that way. Many women with compulsive-eating problems find it excruciatingly painful that others should think that they themselves are large because of the amount they eat. They cannot bear other people making the connection between food intake and body size. This explains, in part, the public side of the compulsive eater who eats sparingly. Other women feel differently. A new and highly publicized method for weight control is a procedure of wiring the jaws together. The women involved in this treatment have been extremely large—well over 250 pounds. While their teeth are braced and wired they subsist on a liquid diet. The braces are loosened once a week so that the teeth can be brushed.

These various ways of coping with the situation, although particularly extreme, capture the desperation that many compulsive eaters experience, and illustrate how compulsive eating is both a very painful activity and one which is enormously hard to give up. When people repeatedly act in a way that causes them a lot of pain we look to the possible reasons that are involved. Labeling such behavior simply as self-destructive, for example, does not increase one's understanding of the forces behind compulsive eating. Instead, it judges the activity negatively and this provides yet another reason for the compulsive eater to adopt a self-deprecating attitude which is relieved only by a binge or yet another timetable to lose the weight. It is our experience that before an habitual activity—in this instance, eating compulsively—can be given up, the reasons for it need to be explored. As I argued earlier, getting fat is a very definite and purposeful act connected to women's social position. Before giving up compulsive eating the meanings of the fat for the individual woman need to be explored. In giving up compulsive eating she is almost certainly going to stabilize at a lower weight. In order to feel at home with this new constant weight, and, more importantly, her smaller size, the compulsive eater needs to understand what her previous interest has been in being overweight and in being preoccupied with food intake. If she can understand how her fat has served her she can begin to give it up.

In this chapter, I shall describe six important steps we take in the groups:

1. To demonstrate that the compulsive eater has an interest in being fat.

2. To show that this interest is largely unconscious.
3. Specific exercises are done to bring this theme to a woman's consciousness.
4. Once this interest in being fat is recognized, the meanings for each individual woman can be explored.
5. Then we ask whether the fat does what it is supposed to do.
6. We help each woman reclaim aspects of herself that she has previously attributed solely to the fat.

Because fatness has such negative connotations in our culture it may be hard to imagine that anyone could have an interest in getting fat.

To be fat means to get into the subway and worry about whether you can fit into the allotted space.

To be fat means to compare yourself to every other woman, looking for the ones whose own fat can make you relax.

To be fat means to be outgoing and jovial to make up for what you think are your deficiencies.

To be fat means to refuse invitations to go to the beach or dancing.

To be fat means to be excluded from contemporary mass culture, from fashion, sports and the outdoor life.

To be fat is to be a constant embarrassment to yourself and your friends.

To be fat is to worry every time a camera is in view.

To be fat means to feel ashamed for existing.

To be fat means having to wait until you are thin to live.

To be fat means to have no needs.

To be fat means to be constantly trying to lose weight.

To be fat means to take care of others' needs.

To be fat means never saying "no."

To be fat means to have an excuse for failure.

To be fat means to be a little different.

To be fat means to wait for the man who will love you despite the fat—the man who will fight through the layers.

To be fat, nowadays, means to be told by women friends that "Men aren't where it's at," even before you have had a chance to know.

Above all, the fat woman wants to hide. Paradoxically, her lot in life is to be perpetually noticed.

These popular conceptions of fatness, while accurate, present an incomplete picture of the compulsive eater's experience. There is also something positive to be gained from being fat that we must explore. I am not suggesting that the desire to be fat is a conscious one. Indeed, I would argue that people are largely unaware of it, and it is not at all easy to discuss this in the abstract. In the groups we do the following exercise to provide us with insight into some of the ways in which fat serves us. I suggest you close your eyes for ten minutes and have someone read you the following fantasy exercise:

Imagine yourself in a social situation... this could be at work, at home, at a party, whatever... notice what you are wearing... whether you are sitting or standing... whom you are talking to, or having something to do with.... Now imagine yourself getting fatter, in the same social situation... you are now quite large.... What does it feel like?... Notice what you are wearing... whether you are sitting or standing.... Notice all the details in this situation... how are you getting on with the people around you?... Are you an active participant or do you feel excluded?... Are you having to make more or less of an effort?... Now see if you can detect any messages that this very fat you has to say to the world.... Is there any way in which you can see it serving you?... Are there any benefits you see from being this fat in this situation?...

When we do this exercise in the groups we get a variety of responses and many are what one might expect. They include feeling like a freak, an outsider, or a blob or assuming that whomever one had contact with was doing so out of pity or was also a freak. But more significantly, people were able to see a new meaning in the fat. For some, the fantasy sparked feelings of confidence and substance as though the fat represented concrete strength. For others, being fat felt very safe as though it were an excuse for failure and that in worrying about body size the women did not have to think about any other possible problems in their lives. Some women felt that being fat protected them insofar as it allowed them to contain their feelings; other women talked of feeling comfortable in their bigness and warmth and having plenty of love to give to others. However, the most common benefits that women saw in being large had to do with a sexual protection. In seeing herself as fat, a woman is often able to desexualize herself; the fat prevents her from considering herself as sexual. Having done the exercise, so many women report feeling relaxed at a party, not feeling they were on show or had to compete but were comfortably talking to female friends. Others felt the fat separated them from the kind of women they had ambivalent feelings about—the ones whom they perceived as self-involved, trivial and vain. Others felt that it meant they could hold their own and keep unwanted intruders away. Many women felt a relief at not having to conceive of themselves as sexual. Fatness took them out of the category of woman and put them in the androgynous state of "big girl."

As people in the groups are slowly able to incorporate these positive aspects and benefits into their views of fatness, they begin to develop a different self-image. The image of fatness then is no longer one-sidedly negative, inextricably tied up with an ugly vision. Instead of regarding themselves as hopeless, helpless or willfully destructive, they can see that their compulsive eating has had some purpose, that it has had a function. As this function becomes more apparent it is possible to be more generous to yourself, to regard the compulsive eating and the attempt to get fat as a way in which you have handled particularly difficult situations. The compulsive eating can then be looked on as an attempt to adapt to a set of circumstances rather than as irrational, "crazy" behavior.

I would now like to explore just why these images of largeness are comforting. What is it that women are saying they feel more capable of when they are fat?

Many women experience the social expectations placed on them as unattainable, unrealistic, undesirable, burdensome and oppressive. Central among these expectations is the feeling that women should be, on the one hand, decorative, attractive and an embellishment to the surroundings and on the other hand, that they should do the hard concrete work of raising the children, running households, while at the same time maintaining jobs outside the home. For many women the physical model of the shy, retiring flower, demurely smiling beneath lowered eyelashes, is too frail and insubstantial to accomplish the daily tasks of living that are their responsibility. As such, to these women the fat represents substance and strength. Harriet, a thirty-five-year-old community worker who lives with her husband and two children, put it this way: "I had the feeling that my fat gives me substance and physical presence in the world. It allows me to do all the things I have to do. In the fantasy I saw myself in my office sitting at my desk and taking up an enormous amount of space. I felt the capacity to do anything I needed to do—challenge my boss and fight more effectively for the community group that I'm there to serve. I felt my strength in this exaggeration of my size. Then in my fantasy I went home, and with the realization of the extra bulk it struck me that I walked into an antagonistic situation with my fat as my armor. As I walk into the house I am reminded of all the tasks that have to be done there that I either execute personally or direct others to do. I feel quite angry about all this, both about feeling so bossy but, of course, also because the terrain of the household is mine—and not by choice. So I see the fat in the situation as making me feel like a sergeant major—big and authoritative. When I go through this fantasy seeing myself thin, what immediately strikes me is just how fragile and little I feel, almost as though I might disappear or be blown away."

Barbara, a twenty-seven-year-old book-jacket designer, talked about the annoying expectations of many of her male colleagues. She felt that her bulk and substance was an expression of her need to be noticed as a productive human being rather than a decorative accompaniment to the environment. She felt that whenever she looked the slightest bit sexy—and this corresponded to the way she looked when she was thin—her colleagues only reacted to the sexual aspect of her. She experienced this as both a frightening demand and also a deflection from her work. As it is for so many women, taking her work seriously was quite a struggle for Barbara. She had grown up with the idea that she would work for a couple of years after school and then get married and have children. But ideas had changed and by the time she left college she wanted to work to have a career rather than for a stop-gap measure. This decision was not trivial; she felt she had a lot of support for her change of mind because all her friends were also pursuing work as a central part of their lives. But Barbara was in conflict about her capacity to be a good worker, not because her art work was erratic, second-rate or inadequate but because she was battling with an unconscious idea

that taking herself seriously in her work life was
inappropriate. In the group we were able to expose
this conflict and Barbara saw how difficult it was for
her to be thin/sexual on the job because she and the
men there collaborated in trivializing her. She felt
the only way she could hold on to that aspect of
herself that was involved in a career was by having
an extra layer covering her femaleness. As she said,
"The fat made me one of the boys."

In the group we also worked to expose the
conflict that Barbara felt about the different models
of adult female behavior; the one she grew up with
which was modeled not only on her mother's life but
also on a popular conception of femininity in the
1950s and early 1960s; and a model that she and her
contemporaries were struggling to articulate, a view
of womanhood that was less limiting and struck at
the very roots of women's oppression within the
family. This conflict is, in my experience, a difficult
and painful one for many women and not one that
will be resolved by a sudden flash of insight. In the
groups it is important to realize that the goal is not
necessarily to resolve this or any other conflict
which may lie at the root of the compulsive eating.
What is important, however, is that the conflict be
brought to light, that the woman should understand
that it exists and that eating compulsively is not
going to make it go away—it may cover it. The fat
may provide for something less threatening to
worry about. But the critical issue is to make the
woman acknowledge the conflict so that it need not
be expressed indirectly and hidden from the person
who is experiencing it. This acknowledgment then
becomes a powerful weapon in the fight against
compulsive eating. It is very reassuring to discover

that there are substantial reasons for why one is eating in such a seemingly inexplicable way. It provides one with the tools; thus when Barbara, for instance, noticed that she was bingeing, she could ask herself what was really troubling her. If she did not come up with any spontaneous answer she could review her day or events leading up to the binge and see if there were any incidents that particularly encapsulated her conflict about who she could be as a woman in the world. In this way she could decode her own behavior. This then gave her a chance to intervene on her own behalf and she could move on to ask herself whether being fat in that particular situation was really going to help her out.

So one meaning of the fat is the woman's need for recognition in a work setting. But another theme that frequently comes up is almost diametrically opposed to this. It is often the case that people's fat fantasies are widely different and that even within the same person the fat may express many different meanings. Barbara, for example, could see the use of the fat in her attempt to be taken seriously at work, but at the same time we discovered her fat also symbolized her fear of being successful both in work and courtship. Her fear of success, of course, stems largely from the social position of a young woman of today growing up with contradictory messages about what she can accomplish. Stepping outside what has been laid out for one is frightening. A useful, protective device is to make the assumption that one will fail; in Barbara's view the excess weight provided her with an excuse should she not succeed in love and work. She found out that she could not bear the idea that her work life or love life would not be satisfying, once she had committed herself to trying to have both. She felt sure that if there were failure on either score, it would be attributable to a character weakness on her part. This idea, in turn, was so painful that she focused instead on her weight as an excuse in the case of potential failure. As long as she was overweight, and love and career did not quite work out as she hoped, she could imagine that if she were thin, everything would be just fine. Thus, this fantasy allowed her to exert some control over her circumstances as though in an inspired weight loss she would be able to sort out social attitudes to women at work and love relationships with men.

In Barbara's case the fat served two distinct purposes, albeit somewhat contradictory ones. Firstly, it provided her with a way to express competence on the job; secondly, if she did not succeed at work or in her love life she could blame her excess weight. As these two themes emerged in the course of her therapy, Barbara was able to see that getting fat was a personal adaptation she had made in trying to cope with a very difficult situation. In addition to being able to expose the conflict, she was able to see the dilemma of a young career woman today and how she felt she had to deny or solve the difficulties facing her entirely on her own. Other women in the group identified with what Barbara was going through and, as they began to share their difficulties, they broke their individual isolation and feelings of impotence which had in part led to the weight gain.

Failure and success are powerful concepts within our world. Very early on we absorb the idea that a limit has been set on what is available and we learn to compete for what is around. If we are successful we are rewarded, and if we are unsuccessful our lot is to suffer. When we are very young it is hard to see quite how the odds are stacked or in whose favor, and the competition seems fair—with failure or success being the individual's fault or triumph. As we get older, we may question the basic assumptions behind the scramble or even how the pie is divided up, whether it is the number of possible "A"s in a class or the division of labor itself. But ideas absorbed and structured into the personality die hard, and feel almost impenetrably lodged. While we may reject the notion of competition because of the devastating effects it has wrought in relationships between people as well as in world politics, we may nevertheless find ourselves unwittingly competitive. Competitive feelings get triggered in a situation of scarcity where there is not enough to go round, or where only a certain number of people can be rewarded. The apprehension of possible exclusion or denial can foster either a desire to compete individually for some of the scarce resource or to sort out cooperatively a way to deal with the shortage. Another alternative is to opt out of the competition. But by and large, as we grow up we are encouraged to compete against others. In school this is expressed through grades or which team you make or your position in class. But girls and boys, women and men, are trained to cope with scarcity and competition in different ways. The cliché of "let the boy win at tennis" expresses an aspect of the competition between women and men. We learn that if there is a game between the sexes in which one side has to lose, we had better make sure we are the losers. In general, men are taught to compete against other men for jobs and status. They gain prestige in the world of work by being better than other men, and they measure their success by comparing it with that of others. Although women also exist in the world of work, men are rarely encouraged to compete against women because they do not tend to take women's presence in traditional male preserves very seriously. Similarly, women are strongly discouraged from competing with men or each other at work. Woman are forced to compete with each other for the man who will help the winner secure her social position. A woman's success in the world continues largely to be regarded as a reflection of her husband's status. In this battle for social survival, women are essentially competing on the basis of their sexual appeal while other aspects of their personality are viewed as attributes to be paraded in the attempt to secure a man.

Women's liberation is challenging this value system for both women and men. However, those of us in our twenties and upward have grown up with these values and ideas and, although they are being shaken up, they nevertheless continue to play a significant part in our personalities. Often we do not realize how much a part of us they are. When we do notice these competitive feelings, we find them distasteful and inappropriate in a changing world and try to suppress, hide or ignore them.

The acknowledgment of a whole range of competitive feelings is difficult for many women and often we attempt to cover these feelings by getting fat. The fat has several functions in this regard.

1. It provides space and protection for the feelings. Without the fat a woman might worry unconsciously that her feelings will be exposed. There would be no difficulty in getting thin if the competitive feelings could find no place to hide and just disappeared. But problems like that never do just disappear; they either get actively repressed and reappear in another form; or they become exaggerated and completely exposed; or they get acknowledged with the potential for being worked through.

2. The feeling of being fat-outsize—larger than life, removes the possibility of competing since everyone knows that "fat women can't win and, in fact, aren't even in the same game."

3. In the very act of compulsive eating—the most frequent route to getting fat—one may be attempting to blot out competitive feelings that may have been stirred up. Again, we see the dual function of compulsive eating—to dull the feeling that is difficult to cope with and to provide a way for the energy behind the worry (in this case feeling competitive) to be harnessed to a more familiar concern about body size.

Compulsive eating also helps out in other circumstances when women are frightened to show certain emotions. These are feelings such as anger, that women are afraid to show because they are considered inappropriate for women, many of whom have been hurt when they expressed them.

A preparation for a life of inequality inevitably leads to many of these turbulent and hence socially unacceptable feelings in women. In addition to difficulties with competition in which women are expected to lose on all fronts except the sexual one where she must succeed in getting her man in order to move toward adulthood, other feelings engendered by social situations can be swallowed up by the fat.

Anger is a particularly difficult emotion for women to accept in themselves. Jennifer is a forty-eight-year-old teacher in London. She is married and has two sons, aged eighteen and twenty. Professionally competent and well recognized for her work in inner-city education, she has had a history of compulsive eating since she got married. Jennifer was an orphan, brought up by many different foster parents. She never felt safe or loved in any of the homes in which she stayed and at eighteen she received a scholarship to college and left her last foster parents permanently. At that point she was truly on her own with no pretense that anyone around her was taking care of her. She felt quite strong and able to cope, and remembers feeling particularly relieved that she did not have to pretend to be grateful for every ounce of attention paid to her. She roomed with other young women and felt quite envious of their family life. When she was twenty-five she got married to Doug, a draughtsman, and for the first time found herself in a stable family environment. Jennifer decided to work for a couple of years so that they would feel more secure financially. It was at that time Jennifer noticed that she was becoming preoccupied with her food intake, and her weight began to fluctuate wildly. Jennifer knew that psychological issues often got expressed in weight gain or loss but just could not pinpoint what was going on because she felt that for the first time her life was making some kind of sense and she felt a security that she had not thought possible before. Both of her pregnancies proceeded relatively comfortably. Jennifer took four years off from her work as a teacher and then went for further training before resuming a full-time job. The family stayed in the same neighborhood for twenty years and Jennifer developed some solid friendships and, as she put it, "a real feeling of community." Yet she continued to eat in a way she found quite disagreeable, alternately picking and shoveling. The only way she could understand this behavior was by seeing it as an expression of how inadequate she felt her own parenting had been. She saw herself continuing the previous pattern of erratic caring of herself. This insight provided her with some relief but the eating problem still continued. In the course of her therapy, we did a fantasy of Jennifer fat and thin with her foster parents in the same room. In a response to a question about what the fat was saying to her many foster parents, Jennifer was suddenly overcome by enormous feelings of rage. She experenced the fat as all the poisonous, venomous feelings she had stored up through the many years of being shuffled about. She felt that if the fat itself had a mouth it would shriek hateful and angry thoughts to all those people who had supposedly cared for her. Her fat was a way to keep quiet about all those feelings but she also experienced it as an indictment of the inadequate parenting she had had. As we discussed it more, she said that without it nobody would know that she had suffered and people would take it for granted that she could just float through life quite easily, that she was like everyone else. Once she had felt these feelings of rage much of her compulsive eating made sense. She began to notice that whenever she felt angry, with her kids, at school or with Doug, she rushed to eat to swallow the feelings.

To feel the anger was to put herself in jeopardy—she felt a tape going through her head every time she got angry, it said: "Nice girls don't. Be grateful or you'll be thrown out." These sentences were those that were taught to her very early on indeed. To express anger or disappointment in a foster home was unacceptable and carried with it not only this exclusion from the female sex but also the fear of abandonment and rejection. If she got angry at her foster parents she would be sent back. The discovery of the roots of the compulsive eating eased the situation for Jennifer. She began to allow herself to experience anger directly and risk the consequences instead of eating it away. She also became aware of her anxiety about levels of insecurity she felt within her own family as though if she expressed displeasure at something she would be turfed out. On most levels she felt quite safe with Doug and it was, in fact, this safety that had allowed that historic anger and rage to emerge—albeit indirectly—in the first place. Jennifer was caught in a changing situation. As a youngster she had to put up and shut up. She could show no anger or rebellion. When she was able to leave these unsatisfactory homes and start her own family she felt more secure and in charge of the situation but she understandably carried past insecurities with her. The part of her that felt securely established with Doug, her career and the kids provided enough space for her to reject the dreadful past she had had but she was not quite able to do that openly and expressed that rejection by eating compulsively.

In Jennifer's case, her fat was a delayed response to a series of extremely precarious and deprived home circumstances. It was not until she had set up her own home that she found herself eating erratically and yoyo-ing on the scales. This pattern—becoming obsessively involved with food after the troublesome events have passed—is quite common. There seems to be a psychological mechanism that works in the following way for some people: a girl grows up in a difficult environment, but needs to survive it as much intact as possible in order to get out. Any expression of breakdown or weakness would only prolong the imprisonment and make escape more difficult. All her resources are harnessed so that she can endure the horrible circumstances and prepare for an exit. She finally leaves this setting and puts herself in a safer place. As she begins to relax in her new-found safety and lets her defenses down all the wretched feelings from the past have a chance to come up. It is not as though in leaving the situation she has left the feelings behind. The safety and security of the new situation provides for a detoxification process. But these feelings are very powerful and very often extremely painful and the human organism may respond by trying to continue to ward them off. In the case of someone who starts compulsive eating at this point, what is happening is that the feelings are coming up but are experienced as too dangerous to confront. The woman turns to compulsive eating to anesthetize the feelings and cover them with a layer of fat. The feelings do not get expressed and cleansed; instead they get transformed into a symptom which then has to be demystified before it can be made to go away.

I should now like to discuss why the expression of anger is so difficult for women. In Jennifer's case, there was an explicit threat of expulsion should she express anger at her treatment but in general, women are actively discouraged from expressing anger, rage, resentment and hostility. We are raised to be demure and accept what we are given with no complaints. We all learn how little girls are made of sugar and spice and all things nice. So we try hard not to show our anger or even feel it ourselves. When we rebel and show dissatisfaction we learn we are nasty and greedy. Whether we realize it or not we are being taught to accept silently a second-class citizenship. Secondary status is further compounded by having our anger denied us. Anger provides a way for people to challenge injustices at whatever level—be it a child's anger in response to a punitive parent or the collective anger of others fighting to have their day-care centers restored.

But there are few models of righteously angry women for us to follow. Indeed, I think most of us are pretty frightened around an angry woman—so unfamiliar is the sight. Anger, as a legitimate emotion for many women, has no cultural validation. Little girls are encouraged to cry if they do not get what they are wanting instead of angrily protesting; "There, there, dear." In Edward Albee's play *Who's Afraid of Virginia Woolf*, Martha, the angry wife who protests against the life of a helpmate, is portrayed as a bitch and a harridan. Much of popular culture attests to the negative value we place on women's rage. It is not surprising, therefore, to find that for many women, the unconscious motivation behind the weight gain is a flight from anger. In this case, the symbolic meaning of the fat is a "Fuck you!"

Behind the suppression of anger lies one of the

most important themes for women today. Gaining weight to express anger, to be able to say, "Fuck you," is only a part of a larger problem. Expressing anger is an assertive act. Assertion for women is difficult. Consider these typical situations:

Ann is extremely tired after a long day at work. She plans to spend the evening alone just resting, watching television and reading. Her neighbor Jack calls up and asks if she would not mind helping out by baby-sitting for his children for an hour while he and his wife go to the store. Ann feels she must be cooperative but knows from past experience that the hour is rarely such and the whole evening will be gone. Reluctantly, she goes next door. At 11:30 p.m. Jack and Penny return. They have been to the store and the movies. Ann is at this point angry but blames herself for having agreed to baby-sit without conditions in the first place. She goes home muttering to herself and eats.

Bill and Roz planned to go to the movies together. Bill calls Roz up from work to check that it will be alright for him to bring some friends home to dinner. Roz, who had already started cooking, takes his decision as a *fait accompli* and reluctantly agrees, feeling she has no right to refuse. She goes into the kitchen and starts banging around fixing dinner and feeling very moody. She assumes that Bill has forgotten about their movie date and she feels rejected. She feels put upon as she is cooking but also feels guilty for being so ungenerous and unspontaneous. She noshes her way through the cooking and when Bill and his friends sit down for supper she shovels the food into her mouth, at this point angry about her inability to assert herself in the first place.

In both situations Ann and Roz feel unentitled to demand what they actually want. Ann is afraid to set limits on her own altruism and Roz does not stand up for herself and the movie date. Both women blame themselves for not having asserted themselves and also for feeling selfish enough even to conceive of their own wants in the first place. They both eat away the bad feelings and focus the negative feelings on the food rather than addressing the difficult issue of assertion. *They feel safer using their mouths to feed themselves than using them to talk and be assertive. They imagine that their fat is making the statement for them while the suffering prevents the words from coming out.* None of this is conscious, the seeds for this behavior have been planted in the mother-daughter relationship in which the mother encourages the girl child to adopt a pleasing manner. The mother prepares her daughter for a life in which major decisions are made for her rather than by her. *The girl will be taught to accept that her needs come second and that keeping quiet is safer than assertion.* Consequently, women are confused and afraid to act on their own behalf. To do so often makes one appear aggressive and *that* has such negative connotations for women that it feels less dangerous to adopt an acquiescent stance. So for women, there is great confusion between unassertive, assertive and aggressive behavior. The recent rush of courses and self-help assertion-training books is witness to the magnitude of this problem. And there have been unfortunate consequences for women who have risked stepping out of line in the past. *Women have been condemned as castrating or domineering when they have attempted to assert their rights.*

There are, in addition, other consequences about being unassertive that add to the problem. If one is not trained to be assertive it is quite hard to define how much you will or will not give to others. By and large, women are taught to nurture the world. As one psychoanalyst, Mercy Heatley, put it, women are the "sewage treatment plants" for the family and, as such, are always giving emotionally to others. In discussing what their fat and food symbolized to them many women have described it as being a kind of "fuel for the furnace," a private storehouse they can draw on when they need to be replenished in order to go on feeding others. For some women, however, the fat in this case represents a rejection of just this kind of service to others. In the woman's mind the excess weight is a message to others to keep away and not make any demands, almost a "Can't you see I've got enough on my hands without worrying about anyone else." For others, it is a statement which embodies both these feelings—the fat expresses a shapeless capacity to both absorb and repel outside demands. So the fat expresses both an attempt to be separate from others while, at the same time, a woman's sheer size encompasses everything around her. It is as though the woman can take on everyone else's needs without them actually penetrating her—the weight acts as a shock absorber for others and as a cushion against her becoming too affected.

As I have said in discussing responses to the fat fantasy, the most frequently stated advantage women saw in being fat had to do with sexual

protection. It is almost as though through the
protective aspects of the fat, women are saying they
must deny their own sexuality in order to be seen as
a person. *To expose their sexuality means that
others will deny them their personhood.* In adolescence, girls are supposed to magically transfer their
friendship interest in boys to a sexual one—they
learn a ritual called dating. This sudden transition
can be quite formidable and difficult to cope with.
As Mary, a twenty-seven-year-old doctor, put it,
"When I was about six or seven years old, girls and
boys used to play together. Then we were separated
out and, until the age of eleven, contact with boys
was fairly limited, particularly as I went to an
all-girls school during that period. Then at twelve I
went to a coed junior high school and looked
forward to playing with the boys again. Their games
seemed more exciting and I really missed the
adventures they got up to. However, something
weird seemed to be happening; instead of fooling
around together we were supposed to fix ourselves
up real pretty and accumulate dates. This was a way
for us to continue to hang out with the guys. But
along with this went a whole series of rules and
regulations about kissing and touching—it seemed
to me as if in order to play with the fellows I had to
put out. This was quite disconcerting, not because I
didn't like kissing, which I did, but because it
seemed that all of a sudden girls and boys were
really different and had to relate to each other
within a rigid set-up. It was really quite confusing
for all of us and everything seemed downhill from
there on. Sports were divided and we had the great
job of cheering the boys on. I kept feeling that if this
is going to be what being grown up is all about I'll

keep my puppy fat on and try and avoid this whole dating trip."

So Mary spent the next fifteen years, as she put it, "slightly overweight." She noticed during the course of her therapy that her eating binges occurred almost uniformly when she was in any kind of potentially sexual situation. She would gorge away before going to a party, for instance, and convince herself that she was too big to be considered sexual. This allowed her a kind of ease to relate to people at the party—women and men—on her terms rather than on the exchange value of her body. The example of Mary shows quite clearly how the fat is conceived as providing a means of removal from the sexualizing and hence, also competitive aspects of relationships for women.

This sexual division has wide-ranging consequences. Many women have shared the feeling that being fat was a way to stand out in a crowd, to be noticeable, to be different without having to invest as much as they assume thin, attractive women do.

Several women have mentioned that their sex was a disappointment to their parents. Rita remembers eating energetically in order to get big, to prove her existence. Quite strikingly, she stopped bingeing for the first time when she got pregnant. When she had life inside her she felt this was ample evidence of her right to exist. If Rita could reproduce, she had a real role, as a mother, even if she had felt unwanted as a child.

These varied explanations of the meanings behind the fat, from eating as protection to eating as an expression of anger, will not necessarily provide they key for everyone who feels they have this problem. Because the syndrome of compulsive eating, compulsive dieting, weight loss and weight gain is so highly developed and, in a sense, so absorbing a preoccupation in itself, it may be hard to get outside it enough to realize just what it is doing for you. In a sense, compulsive eating provides a beautiful, insulated world: obsessing about how terrible you are for overeating leads to feelings of self-disgust; these feelings have no outlet and are quickly covered up or numbed by the intake of food or banished by the fantasy of reincarnation after the plan for the new diet has been made. All negative feelings get harnessed to complaints and self-loathing about body size and eating habits and the fat provides a less threatening issue to worry about than other possible problems. It may also be true that while the fat has one meaning for you today, it has had quite another when it originally developed. In other words, the historic reasons and driving force behind the impulse to get fat in the first place may be quite different from its current significance, so it often proves useful to look back and see how getting fat has helped people at certain times in their lives. In order to tap this information in the groups we do weight histories to reveal when the "problem" first started. I should like to illustrate this point by drawing on some case histories of women I have worked with. Some of the historic reasons that I will outline will be of clearly feminist content and others will be less explicitly so, though in each example it will be obvious what feminine personality-development has meant to each of the women whose lives I am describing.

Rea was an only child. Her parents had high expectations for her which included academic excellence, sociability and beauty. She felt pressed by these demands to be the perfect, happy child and felt that she did not have much space in which to develop her own independence. She became quite overweight in adolescence and it was to this period that we returned to examine when she came into therapy in her early thirties. Her fat began to make sense set against the background of intense parental concern that she be successful. Rea did not see herself in the same light as did her parents. She felt inadequate. She felt that she was a selfish, ungrateful and bad person. She felt that she could not cope with her parents' demands and that she would be increasingly incompetent. Her fat expressed both the resentment at having to be so perfect and the need to hide and contain the bad person she felt she was inside. She feared being thin because she felt she would then be everything her parents wanted; she would be in their image and without a self.

Jane, a fifty-five-year-old legal secretary, put on weight after her mother's death. Up to the age of twenty-five, Jane had been quite thin and fairly relaxed about her body image. She was an only child, her father died when she was a teenager and she was very close to her mother. She married when she was twenty-two but shortly afterward her husband Tom was sent overseas to fight in World War II. When her baby girl Carol was eighteen months old Tom returned from the war. About a year later Jane's mother died of cancer. For the preceding year and a half she had been losing a lot of weight and looked very thin and ill. When Jane officially stopped mourning she began to put on weight. By the time she was twenty-seven she was 25 to 30 pounds heavier than she had ever been before, except during her pregnancy. She was quite staggered by the increase in her size and at first she put it down to lack of exercise after Carol's birth. Friends suggested that maybe she had enjoyed pregnancy so much that her excess weight was a desire to look continually pregnant. But this explanation made little sense to Jane because her pregnancy had not been the easiest time for her. A psychiatrist friend at the time expounded that she wanted to look pregnant so she could get the attention and praise from Tom he assumed she had missed at the time of her genuine pregnancy. The weight stayed on and eventually, as standards in fashion and health demanded slimness, Jane started the round of diets and diet doctors. Outwardly Jane had a fairly contented home life—she and Tom really liked each other and Carol, their only child, kept up continued contact with them after she had grown up and left home. However, Tom reported that almost every night Jane cried out in her sleep for *her* mother. In the course of therapy this piece of information from Tom was discussed in detail. Jane came to understand that the weight gain had much to do with the loss of her mother, as she said, "My mother died tragically of cancer. She became very thin before her death. I've had a need to feel big ever since then and worried, I suppose, that if I get thin I might disappear or die like her." Facing her mother's death and her own fears about dying if she became thin allowed Jane to determine a size for herself that was both physically and psychologically comfortable. As it turned out, Jane felt that she no longer wished to be as svelte as she imagined she might and her weight stabilized at about fifteen pounds lower than it had been.

Death has been a factor in the fat for other women with whom I have worked. Sheila, a twenty-eight-year-old graduate student, had lost her older brother Ivan when he was twelve and she was ten. She gained weight from that time on and in the group we discovered that the origin of becoming fat had had two distinct symbolic meanings. Sheila felt the oversized body allowed her to carry her brother with her. She remembered that she had really enjoyed being with him and played with him a lot. Ivan had been the pride and joy of the family, first born and male it was anticipated that he would fulfill his parents' ambitions. About two years after his death they had another child, Maureen. Sheila felt a great deal of responsibility for being both a little mother to Maureen and a son to her parents. To her, what a son meant was quite distinct from what being a daughter had meant. It demanded that she be very good at sports, achieve scholastically and plan for a successful career of which her parents could be proud. In being a daughter she was expected to do decently at school but a career was to come second to a successful love life. In her adolescence, Sheila's father took her to ball games. She enjoyed being one of the boys and having a much more developed relationship with her father than she had had before she became a teenager. In the therapy, what emerged was a guilt for feeling good that she could have so much of her father. She imagined that if her brother had lived, this would not have been the case. Symbolically, she felt the second meaning of her fat was to round out her curves—to make her less feminine so she could look

more the part of a son. When she had lost weight
over the years she took with her the same desire to
look boyish and she was always annoyed that she
still had hips and breasts and could not achieve the
androgynous body she wanted.

Sheila had been trying to cope with the problem
of how to be the teenage son and the little mother.
This latter aspect is one showed by many girls at
even earlier ages than Sheila. Often a seven-year-old
daughter will be expected to be mother's little helper
or substitute in looking after the babies that follow
her.

Melinda, the eldest girl in a family of seven,
recalls a blissful early childhood when she and her
older brother would play together. When she was
seven years old her mother had another baby. It
seemed to Melinda that her childhood was over; not
only did she have to share her mother with yet
another child but she was expected to, and indeed
did, carry out many grown-up tasks. As more and
more babies came, Melinda became a second
mommy to them so that at eighteen when she left
home she felt well trained to start her own family.
She became large instead, however, explaining that
if she looked like a big earth mother no one would
assume she was at all available. She had had her lot
for the moment!

This mothering learned so early on leads many
women to teach their daughters to deprive and deny
themselves. Florence and her daughter Laura both
had compulsive eating problems. Florence's ideology was that eating goodies was an indulgence—
and a disgusting one at that. She felt it was indecent

to give into oneself with almost any form of pleasure, but particularly bodily pleasures. Food and sex were inviting and exciting but one must stay away from them. Florence ate sparingly all year round. On vacation when she overate she felt guilty and on her return would immediately put herself on the Mayo Clinic Diet to lose the excess. She was iron-willed and very self-controlled but terribly afraid of food. Her husband hid his candies in the glove compartment of his car and she considered his love of dessert a sign of his character weakness. Laura rebelled against this code of self-denial. She despised her mother's meanness with herself and characterized her as compulsively thin. She felt her mother never gave herself pleasure with food or sex. Laura chose the opposite route and tried to get pleasure from both activities. However, since the food and sex were both experienced behind closed doors with one ear open for her mother's intrusions, Laura could not be as much in control as she wanted and her eating expressed these tensions. In the group, she learned to eat just for herself and her own pleasure without having to get so big as though to prove her mother was right. She did not have to be ostracized by her size in order to give to herself.

Because of the prevailing position of women in the family, mothers also deny themselves in situations where there just is not enough to go round. They make sure that in a situation of shortage their husbands and children have as much as possible. If a mother fails to provide enough food on the table she feels herself a failure. When prices soar, a mother with a fixed income has less and less to spend on the family shopping and even though she experiences this along with all other house-keepers, it is she alone who must face the family and the complaints and disappointment if the food is not up to scratch. In the depression of the 1930s this was particularly acute; money was very scarce and there was never enough food on the table. Mothers talking about this period say they held back so there would be enough for the rest of the family—they could always make do, *they* were not at school using their brains or out on the streets looking for work everyday, so they felt it was only right that they should suffer.

Carolyn, one of the daughters of that time who subsequently became fat, said, "When I was young it was depression time. My mother would go hungry and try to be sure to provide enough food for us kids, which there wasn't. When I got married I had enough food for the first time in my life and I feel like I'm eating to protect myself against those terrible feelings of hunger I had as a child."

Rose, Carolyn's daughter, born at the end of the Second World War, remembers battles she had with her mother who worried lest she not eat enough—she recalled all the spoonfuls she ate for the poor starving children in Europe, never understanding how eating extra would help them.

Rose remained quite slender until the age of seventeen when she left home to travel round Europe. When she returned, her parents greeted her with approval about her gain in weight. She, however, was quite unhappy being that big—she felt it made her too like them. She got involved with the diet-binge syndrome for the next twelve years. The following themes were explored in her therapy. When she had lived at home, a way to rebel against her parents had been to be thin. Not only were both her parents overweight but they also constantly encouraged her to eat. When she left home, she gained weight as an expression of her conflict about giving up her parents. The fat was a way to take with her a part of her home life—her parents. One of the most critical parts of her therapy was the termination process. Rose had at this point lost about twenty-five pounds and stabilized at a weight she felt fitted her frame. The anticipated separation from the therapist and from the fat brought forth issues related to Rose's childhood struggles to separate herself from her mother. For Rose, these battles about food symbolized her attempts to strike out on her own, to define herself and develop some independence from her mother. As the conflict was brought to light—that is, both Rose's interest in developing a separate identity and her fear of it because of the social and psychological dangers she perceived if she were separate from her mother—she could feel a safety for the first time in determining her own food intake. Her body for her then expressed this surer feeling of independence; it was defined and self-contained and not "all fat, stuck like a mayonnaisey glue to my mother."

Body size means different things to different women. In Rose's case being large was being stuck, capitulating, it meant accepting all those extra spoonfuls of food she had not wanted; in Barbara's case it was an attempt to desexualize herself in the face of her work colleagues; for Harriet it represented strength and substance; for Jane, her anger, and so on. Not only will fat have different meanings for different women but at different times the meanings will take on more, or less, significance.

At the beginning of a compulsive-eating group a woman may only be able to see the fat as a graphic symbol of everything she dislikes in herself. She may describe it as the ghastly manifestation of the ugliness and horridness she feels inside. The fat both covers and exposes her perceived terribleness. As the group goes on in time and other women share their stories, this same woman may well be able to separate that fat from a definition of ugliness and explore some of the ways her fat has served her in the past. She will be able to see that the fat was an attempt to take care of herself under a difficult set of circumstances. As she moves toward a conscious acceptance of this aspect of the fat she can utilize the self-protective impulse in a different way. As she is able to understand that she became fat as a response—to mother, to society, to various situations—she can begin to remove the judgment that it was good or it was bad. *It just was.* It is extremely painful and difficult, if not impossible, to change if one has a negative self-image. An understanding of the dynamics behind getting fat can help remove the judgment. When the judgment is given up and you can accept that the fat just was, you can go on to the question of, "Is it serving me well now?"

It is necessary for those who work in the area of the unconscious to explain about the existence of an unconscious life which has its own force and symbols. These symbols then need to be translated into the language of everyday experience so that we can explore them. Then, as conscious people, we need to intervene to question the rational and seemingly irrational fears and fantasies that rise from the land of dreams and motives. I find myself in a situation where I have asked the reader to consider that compulsive eating is linked to an unconscious desire to get fat. I have further argued that in order to give up the fat this motivation must be exposed. I will now propose, however, that the protective function the fat is meant to serve is one step away from the truth—that the fat itself does not actually do the job it is meant to do. By attrituting to the fat a powerful protective role, a woman sets herself up for a situation in which a life without the fat would be a defenseless one. This is a frightening proposition indeed. We aim to offer the compulsive eater another option, that of seeing that the qualities she feels are in the weight are, instead, characteristics that she herself possesses but has assigned to the fat. In drawing on various aspects of the histories of women with whom I have worked, I have suggested that the discovery of the meaning of the fat has subsequently led to a reappraisal of whether it is the fat *itself* which actually keeps people away, desexualizes one, helps contain the angry, (hurt, disappointed) feelings or provides substance. If, indeed, it is not the fat itself that has done all these things but rather the individual, two questions arise:

1. How and why has the individual woman withheld this power from herself and attributed it solely to the fat?
2. How can she reappropriate this power so that she feels it to be more a part of her essential self—who she is? This is so that when she gives up the weight she is not giving up the main methods in which she has dealt with the world.

The first question speaks to an issue of crucial importance that arises from the socialization of women. Women are systematically discouraged from taking responsibility for various activities, actions, even thoughts. Men both act for them and describe their experience. While women's experience is exceedingly rich, it is rarely described or heard. Only in literature have women consistently had a voice and a wide audience. In the areas in which women, almost without exception, have taken enormous responsibility—in child-rearing, nurturing and housekeeping—their actions are not seen as defined and delineated because they are described as natural and inevitable. If it is natural you must do it. If it is natural it does not count. Hence it is devalued. Now the paradox lies in the fact that so many of the women described in this chapter have, in fact, defied this stereotype of femininity. They have purposefully gone out into the world and taken on responsibilities that fall outside the scope of their role expectations. But they are caught in a sense of self which denies their power and this self-devaluation seems inexplicable unless it is considered as a consequence of living in a culture that has withheld social power from women and demonstrates this by denying and punishing those who violate prescribed social roles. It is not hard to see how a woman might adopt a self-image that is in tune with the idea that women are powerless. In doing so she accustoms herself to the idea that it is not *her* who has direct power but her "unowned" fat. If it is *her* who can keep people away and not simply her fat then she becomes more in charge of herself. If she is more in charge of herself and acts more for herself in a determined way, will what she wants be attainable? Or will she be punished and rejected by others for daring to define herself rather than fitting in with others' expectations of herself? A further paradox is encapsulated in the compulsive eater whose imagined sense of herself thin is as the powerfully attractive sexual woman. As she subscribes to the image of the thin, sexual woman—a view offered to her consistently by the mass media—she reaches for the elusive power that this image promises but does not deliver. It is precisely this non-recognition of the person in the thin sexual image that causes her unconsciously to reject this thinness. For many women, "thin= sexy=powerful" is an experience that lasts no more than the fleeting moment when she makes her entrance, her initial impact. After that, her image is appropriated by others and translates into "thin= sexy=powerless" and at the same time she may find no way to handle being thin, sexy and in charge. It is this critical question of how women can define and manage their own sexuality that is being grappled with so often in the fat/thin dilemma. And it is the lack of support for a redefinition that compounds the woman's relinquishing her *own* power to her fat. This, then, is an explanation both for the occurrence of a symptom and its tenacity. Giving up a symptom and owning the power assigned to it means you are taking yourself seriously. Taking themselves seriously has been a risky business for women. It is helpful to remember here that in both the attempt to conform to appropriate female behavior and the attempt to reject it, women pay heavily. The issue that confronts us is whether we will risk being punished for rebelling or accept being punished for following feminine roles. As many women have pointed out, the very words "mother" and "wife" conjure up self-denial while the alternative images

of women—career woman, single parent, lesbian—
provoke hostility and ostracization.

Having described the conventions by which
women have been forced to exist I think it clarifies
why we might choose something else—the fat—to
act for us. Reappropriation of your power (temporarily given to the fat) involves a reevaluation of
yourself. This very reevaluation produces a change
in consciousness and with the awareness of what has
been given away, we can slowly incorporate into our
new self-image what belongs to us. In owning the
power of the fat we can give it up.

What is thin about for the compulsive eater?

We know that every woman wants to be thin. Our images of womanhood are almost synonymous with thinness. If we are thin we shall feel healthier, lighter and less restricted. Our sex lives will be easier and more satisfying. We shall have more energy and vigor. We shall be able to buy nice clothes and decorate our bodies, winning approval from our lovers, families and friends. We shall be the woman in the advertisements who lives the good life; we shall be able to project a variety of images—athletic, sexy or elegant. We shall set a good example to our children. No doctors will ever again yell at us to take off the excess weight. We shall be admired. We shall be beautiful. We shall never have to be ashamed about our bodies, at the beach, in a store trying to buy clothes or in a tightly packed automobile. We shall be light enough to sit on someone's knee and lithe enough to dance. If we stand out in a crowd it will be because we are lovely, not "repulsive." We shall sit down in any position comfortably, not worrying where the flab shows. We shall sweat less and smell nicer. We shall feel good going to parties. We shall be able to eat in public without courting disfavor. We shall not have to make excuses for liking food.

These images and desires bombard our consciousness daily. In seeing ourselves thin, we can all find something positive with which to identify. When we are fat we crave thinness as we crave the food, searching within it for the solution to our varied problems.

But the fact is that while many of us want to be thin many millions of women are overweight or concerned with body size. One of the theses of this book is not obvious. Women fear being thin; fat has its purposes and advantages. Our experience shows that many women are positively afraid of being thin. Woman's conscious experience is of wanting to be thin, but her body size can belie this intention suggesting that in the same way that fat plays an active role in our lives, so thinness is the other side of the coin. Being fat serves the compulsive eater in a protective way; being thin is a fearful state—the woman is exposed to the very things she attempted to get away from when she got fat in the first place.

In trying to absorb this idea, I suggest you close your eyes for two minutes and think about a social situation that you were involved in today. This might have been an incident at work, at the shops or in the home.

Now carefully go over what happened in that particular situation.... Notice what you were wearing... whether you were standing or sitting and how you were getting on with the people around you.... Were you an active participant or did you feel excluded?... Be aware of as many details as possible....

Now imagine yourself thin in exactly the same situation.... Notice particularly what you are wearing and how you feel in your body. Are you sitting or standing?... How are you getting on with the people around you?... Notice particularly if there is a difference in the way you are getting on with others now.... Do you feel more or less included?... Are people wanting different things from you?...

When you have become familiar with the details of the situation, see if you are aware of any negative feelings that being thin engenders in you. Is there anything frightening about being thin in this place?

When women in the groups I work with try this fantasy exercise they are often very surprised at the kinds of things they find out about themselves. After an initial joyful experience of seeing themselves thin they contact feelings and ideas associated with thinness that sound like the following:

1. They feel cold and ungiving.
2. They feel angular, almost too defined, and self-involved.
3. They feel admired to the point of having expectations laid on them. They feel they will not be

able to keep people at bay—particularly those with a sexual interest.

4. They do not know how to cope with their own sexual desires; they feel free to be sexual now but unsure of the implications.

5. They feel they command too much power.

6. They do not know how to define the boundaries around themselves and feel invaded by others' attention because they will not know how to fend it off. They are worried about where they exist in this new admiration.

7. They feel uncomfortable amongst other women who throw competitive glances.

8. They are worried by the need to have everything worked out—to have their lives fit together. They feel there are no longer any excuses for the difficulties they face in their lives. They feel they must give up all the pain that their fat has expressed. They are particularly concerned that when they are thin they will have no room to feel blue, and that no one will see their neediness. It is very important to realize that concern about body size, as reflected by these themes, is a constant preoccupation for women because these images are the only socially acceptable models of feminine behavior.

I should like to take each of these feelings in turn and show why they are such common fears when women do that fantasy exercise.

1. The fear that being thin means to be emotionally cold is a familiar one. We know how very deeply our identities are formed around the model of the woman as a giving, caring person. Experiencing oneself as cold and ungiving is in direct conflict with this very basic notion we learn as little girls. How many of us can comfortably accept that there are aspects of ourselves that reject this giving, nurturing woman? We fear being cold so much because we rarely allow ourselves to show this side of our personalities.

Annie, a fifty-eight-year-old teacher and expectant grandmother, said, "All my life I've striven to create a warm and loving place around me. If I imagine myself thin now, I feel icy and frozen, like an emaciated version of myself. I feel I wouldn't fit into my life. It would be as if I'd stopped being lively, warm and giving which is how I see myself now." Just as we think one candy means we eat the whole roll, so we worry that showing any coldness means we shall be cold people. We are expected to be caring and giving and, furthermore, we expect this from ourselves. So many of our daily relationships center on our capacity to nurture others. To be cold, even temporarily, is virtually to deny our own sexual identity.

2. Being angular and too defined causes problems because we are so used to having our personalities defined for us. By this I mean that we tune our antennae to adjust to others' expectations of us because our social position has discouraged us from forging our own identities.

We are defined to fit the traditional female stereotypes. When we struggle for self-definition, we are met with curiosity, lack of support and even hostility. Diane, a Canadian psychiatrist in therapy for compulsive eating, expressed a common fear. She worried that if she were thin, people would think that she was really only interested in herself

and not in others. If she looked thin and beautiful
(in her mind, the two go together), that would mean
she was vain and self-involved since thinness was
something she had to work hard to attain. Diane felt
her fatness covered her feelings of self-importance;
if she were thin, these feelings would be apparent.
Since Diane's work was to help others, the idea that
she might be so involved with herself horrified her.
Her discomfort was of a kind familiar to many
women. We grow up to be concerned with others
and often feel guilty when we notice that we have
our own needs, desires and concerns which really
come first. For Diane, the dilemma was particularly
acute and she noticed that she stuffed several
cookies down her mouth just before sessions with
her patients. By doing this, she felt she was
accomplishing two things: she ensured that she
remained big—which to her meant being stable and
reliable; and she was preventing herself betraying
her feelings of self-involvement when she was
working with someone. Stuffing down the cookies
she stuffed her feelings.

3. Being admired is also not without its difficulties.
If we are admired when we are thin we often feel that
it is only our bodies that are being appreciated. A
woman's body has been her primary asset; how she
sees it measuring up against the bodies of other
women is an important factor determining how she
feels. How she looks will partly determine her
choice of lovers and husband. It is important that
she makes a good impression with her looks to a
much greater extent than her male counterpart.
This, of course, is a preposterous position—to be
valued on the basis of current fashions of sexual

attractiveness. What about the active, thinking part of us? Thus being thin carries with it worries about whether we shall be regarded as a complete person, rather than simply as a sexual one.

4. The desire to be sexual is double-edged. On the one hand, many women associate thinness with sexual desirability, and they feel more in control of their choice of partners. As thin people they feel it is legitimate to select those in whom they are interested; as overweight people they feel they must wait for the man or woman who will fight through the layers to find the person. On the other hand, many women fear the new-found sexuality that being thin promises. Many feel that they will act on it in ways that are different from their current sexual behavior. One of the worries that comes up time and time again in groups is, "If I become thin and very attractive maybe I'll be turned on to other men apart from my husband and I don't want to jeopardize our relationship." We have so little say over the determination of our sexuality and consequently it is often hard for us to feel, let alone act on, what we want sexually.

One woman I worked with spelled it out this way: "If there is less of me, people will see more of me, I shall be exposed. What will be exposed is my sexuality. Fat, I hide it in cheerfulness and pretend I'm not sexual myself. Thin, I reveal a sexuality that is unformed and feels unfettered because I'm thin so rarely that I don't get used to feeling comfortable with my own sexuality."

Images of female sexuality radiate from billboards, the television and the cinema. Advertisements for cars and tractors often show women draped over the goods. Female sexuality becomes a commodity in the eyes of both men and women.

The significance of this last point produces a further complication. Men's sexual objects are women. However, women's sexual objects are also women for sexuality is normally presented in female images. Therefore women become confused if they do not fit the image that has been set up for them. If a woman does not look like the sexually vital woman in the advertisement or on the fashion page, how dare she be sexual?

But why should thinness prove to be a problem of sexuality? For many, the answer lies in the fact that weight has been experienced as a way to avoid sexuality. While avoiding sexuality is a very painful way to cope, it may, nevertheless, be a safer option for women who fear that thinness is equated with sexual desirability. As with all the fantasies attached to thin, in the groups we work on new ways of saying "no" and "yes" to sexuality so that we can be whatever weight and at the same time still struggle to define our sexual needs. Thus, if fat has been a way of saying "no" to sex we must learn to use our mouths to speak to assert the "no" rather than hoping that the world will magically understand that the food we just put in our mouths was an attempt to say "no." Mouths have two important functions—to allow us to speak and to ingest food. Sometimes compulsive eaters worry that they do not know how to use their mouths in the first of these ways.

5. There are, as well, deeper levels of resistance to being thin. One of the fears many women discover

they associate with being thin is that of feeling too powerful. In our culture, girls from a very early age are taught that their role in life is to be one of helpmate to a potent man. Their own sense of identity will develop from their husbands' positions; they will be the wife and loving mother, and the power behind the man. Girls are consistently discouraged from having power in their own right outside the mothering role. The meaning of being thin for many women is that they will be doing *too* well and will have exceeded their social place.

Power presents women with three interrelated problems: the first stems from cultural images of powerful women; the second from the way little girls are brought up; and the third, from the imagined or real consequences of being powerful. The few well-known examples we have of powerful women have either been equated with destruction, like Helen of Troy or Cleopatra, or they have been coupled with images of emasculated men, like Maggie of *Maggie and Jiggs*.

The all-powerful mother is only powerful *as mother*. Once father reenters the home, he reappropriates his authority from *his wife*. Thus, a little girl learns about power in a very confused way; her mother's power, the female power, is negated by that of her father but her father's power, male power, is generally equated with ruthlessness and competition.

In growing up, the young girl learns how to cope with second-class citizenship. Her mother teaches her to yield to others (as she herself does to her husband) and to expect others to define the shape of her world. Concepts of femininity exclude thinking of oneself as powerful and effective because to a woman, "powerful" means "selfish"—acting for oneself means depriving others.

Women risk social isolation if they become too powerful. If a woman is powerful and can take care of herself, she may worry that she will not need anyone else and that she will become too self-contained and alone. This fear is fostered by the reactions of others. Men frequently react against a woman's attempt to be powerful in her own right—"What she needs is a man."

Women are frequently no more encouraging to those women who try to act on their own behalf. They may feel threatened, jealous or betrayed. Thus if we exceed our social place by first conceiving of ourselves as powerful and then acting as powerful people, we may feel ourselves to be in jeopardy.

Work on this problem is an integral part of the groups. We explore why women have been taught to accept this secondary role and examine the power structure of individual families or school networks.

6. A very complicated fear which women almost invariably experience centers on the question of female boundaries. Psychoanalytic literature is full of references to the problem women have with boundary definition. What is meant by boundaries is the amount of space one takes up in the world—where one begins and where one ends. The reason why boundary issues are so difficult for women has social roots in the development of a feminine psychology. We know that the female role requires the woman to be a nurturing, caring person who gives emotional sustenance to the people around her. She is required to merge her interests

with those of others and seek her fulfillment in adjusting her needs and desires to others—mainly lovers and children with whom she is centrally involved. She is actively dissuaded from developing her autonomy economically and emotionally. Being fat expresses an attempt both to merge with others and, paradoxically, to provide an impenetrable wall around herself. Similarly, many women associate thinness with boundary issues. If the fat has been a way to express her separateness and her space, without it the woman will feel quite vulnerable and defenseless. Maggie, a thirty-eight-year-old clerk, put it this way: "If I don't have all this weight *on me,* people will get in real close and I won't have any control or protection." Drawings perhaps describe how these themes are experienced.

In figure A the woman is fat and experiences her true self as existing somewhere inside the fat. The fat provides physical protection against her believed

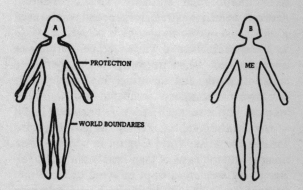

vulnerability. She imagines that if she loses the weight she will be losing a protective coating against the world.

The loss of fixed boundaries of the self produces another of the terrifying states women have associated with loss of weight. This terror a woman may feel is the fear of people invading her. The fat may have allowed her to keep a certain distance from people. She imagines that it all has to do with the fat, that people themselves do not approach her and that she has little right to approach them. Thus, a woman will worry that while thin, people will encroach on her space in an active way and penetrate her. Once again, we see that the body states of fat and thin have been the way that compulsive eaters deal with the difficulties in their social relationships.

7. An issue of enormous difficulty for women is that of competition. They have been forced to compete with each other in order to get the man who will supposedly take care of them and, in particular, to legitimize their sexuality. This competition between women is extremely fierce and painful even if only acted out on an unconscious level. It makes us assess each other so we can feel comfortable or uncomfortable when we engage with others. We walk into parties and unwittingly rank ourselves by our own attractiveness compared with the other women. This is so much a part of our culture that it is even institutionalized. Perhaps its most degraded form is the Miss World Contest in which women compete on the basis of their beauty and personality. Many women attempt to avoid these painful competitive feelings by getting fat. Contemplating a return to thinness exposes the competitive impulses. Many women are not sure how they will cope with

either their own competitive desires or the animosity that they imagine they will rouse in other women.

8. Finally, another of the most frequently expressed fears associated with being thin is crystallized by the statement made by Penny, a twenty-four-year-old teacher. She felt that there were great chunks of her life that had not fallen into place even though she enjoyed her work, friendships and love relationships. She had anticipated that if she could lose ten pounds everything in her life would run smoothly. The reason for this, she felt, was the excess weight. As we probed further together, we discovered that her image of thinness expressed competence and confidence. It allowed no space for anything to go wrong in her life—if she were thin what could possibly be a problem? If she were thin she would not know how to express her pain and sadness if she felt it. She realized that the extra weight provided her with a reason for why everything did not fit into place. Without that reason she worried about her capacity to be in charge of her life in the way that the absorbed media messages promised. As she put it: "If I'm as thin as I really think I want to be I'll just have to get it together!"

Before moving on to detail the actual experience that compulsive eaters have had on the occasions when they have lost weight, it is important to point out that both the images and experiences of thinness contain contradictory messages. The same women attribute divergent worries to fatness and thinness. One might say, "If I'm thin I'll feel weak and almost disappear." Her fat self imagines that the weight gives her strength and substance. We may also discover, however, that for this same woman, thin also connotes a wiry kind of strength and fat its very opposite, a flabby indefinable quality—a blob.

Contradictory images are familiar to all of us in many of our daily activities. It is less commonly understood that the compulsive eater has contradictory feelings about body sizes. Nutritionists, psychologists, doctors and the diet and beauty columns of women's magazines rarely raise the issues that we have found so central in breaking the fat-thin, diet-binge cycle.

It is often the case that compulsive eaters' previous experiences of losing weight and becoming thin have been very difficult. There are many reasons for this which will be explored below but first, some preliminary remarks to provide a context for understanding the varied reasons.

The negative images associated with thinness are largely unconscious. This means that they are not readily accessible to people in their waking lives. The fantasy exercises in this book help to provide clues to finding out more about ideas we hold that we are not generally aware of. Unconscious ideas are as much a force in people's daily existence as the conscious desires, thoughts and actions we put into practice. The unconscious is an active part of all of us and when we attempt to change our behavior or our feelings and it does not work, we look into the varied reasons that stand in our way. Social factors are critical determinants here and must never be underestimated, but our unconscious intent— formed by the repression of socially unacceptable desires—is a persuasive intervener and one that needs to be reckoned with. In addressing the issues of body size and self-image in the groups, we aim to help each other do the emotional work necessary so that this time being thin will be understood in all its ramifications and the anticipated dangers will be minimized. This means that we will be working to:

(1) Explore the ideas that women hold on a conscious and unconscious level about thinness and fatness.

(2) Detach these ideas from body states so that the various qualities an individual ties up with her size will be attributed to her directly and not to her thin self or her fat self. This will allow her to express different aspects of herself without regard to size.

(3) Provide women with alternative ways, apart from eating, by which they can protect, assert and define themselves.

The fears of thinness that compulsive eaters hold based on previous experiences of losing weight center on a number of themes. But the one feeling shared by nearly all compulsive eaters, whatever their own individual psychology, focuses on the effects of losing weight through a diet. Generally, the only way the compulsive eater has found to lose weight has been through a severe restriction of her food intake. Because her body size is such a crucial subject for her, in turning to a diet she invests it with the power to do wondrous things for her. In fact, many women report that once having decided to diet the amount of psychic energy required to actually mobilize, to drastically regulate them-selves—is so enormous that they feel marvelous,

pure, uncriticizable, almost high. Nothing disturbs
them till they break it and the recriminations set in.
Having deified dieting, the breaking of it signals a
return to the tortuous state of compulsive eating.

For a woman the experience of depriving herself
while on a diet operates on two levels. The one
which produces the high allows her to continue the
diet feeling self-righteous and contemptuous of her
previous eating behavior. But on another level,
eating by rules and regulations is a constant
reminder to the compulsive eater that she cannot be
trusted. Thus, when she loses the weight, her
experience of being normal sized and like everyone
else is achieved only at the expense of her remaining
in the prison of compulsive dieting, vigilantly
fighting off the monster of compulsive eating, and
keeping it at bay.

This battle to banish the bingeing puts the
woman in an extremely precarious state. She is as
worried as ever about what can and cannot go into
her mouth and rarely does she feel confident that
this particular diet will end her eating problem. Her
days and nights are no less filled with worries of
food intake and body size. If life for the compulsive
eater is felt to be a process of continuous eating,
then dieting exists outside life and is felt to be
unreal. The addiction continues with all its concomitant obsessions: "Will I be able to resist those
French fries and desserts?" "Will I be able to eat
what Joyce is serving for dinner or will it be too
fattening?" This tension adds to the feeling of
distrust about her capacity to maintain the diet once
the weight has been lost. The specter of hugeness is
always round the corner. The compulsive eater does

not develop a confidence that she will remain thin. She has become a thin woman, someone who looks different and acts in different ways from her fat self, but a new woman whom she does not know very well. She is someone she is not sure she can trust or really get to know because she is unsure of how long she is going to be thin. If she is habitually thin for two months every year having dieted for one month, and fat for the remaining nine, then she is bound to be more familiar with her fat self. She really does not believe that her thin self is going to be around that long so she develops a suspicious relationship with it. Thus, her thin life has a precarious quality which is not conducive to self-confidence.

There is, in addition to all this, a new body to contend with, a smaller version of herself. (We tend to feel so small in our effect on the world, particularly as women, that reducing our physical presence feels almost bizarre.) Connected to this unfamiliarity with her body, is a drastic change in the woman's self-image. Many women report that they wore clothes that were quite unusual for themselves, not simply in the size that the label read, but also in the style that they had selected. Losing weight had held out the promise of fulfilling those aspects of dress they had denied themselves fat. This, for example, may have meant dressing attractively, a taboo idea for most overweight women. "If I am fat, I must be horrible and don't deserve to have nice clothes."

Having dressed in a different way when thin, these women acted differently with others but discovered that they were ill-equipped to deal with the reactions they stirred up. Kate, an anthropology graduate student, discovered that once, when thin, she had been to a party in tight blue jeans and a cheesecloth shirt (in place of her usual cover-up dress over pants) and her women friends, while initially complimentary and supportive, seemed to hover around when their husbands and lovers approached her. Kate was nervous that the other women felt jealous and would dislike her, but she did not know how to keep their husbands away. In the group, we discussed the various meanings of this new clothing. In the end, she was determined that the next time she lost weight, she would risk feeling good and sensual in her clothes without threatening her friends. She decided to share her new and fragile acceptance of her body with her friends and she reassured them that she was not interested in their lovers. This also helped her clear up her own confusion about dressing sensually and sexually.

Body image and protection are very important. In the groups we try to address these two problems in the following ways: group members are encouraged to accept the physical aspects of being fat. Self-acceptance is the key task in the group; without it weight loss and breaking the addiction can only be temporary. We aim for a situation in which women can actually experience the ownership of their fat and the diverse meanings they have attributed to it. When they lose weight they can take its significance with them as necessary. They will not feel that they are losing a protective covering, they grow into their bodies and then they will feel that they have their whole bodies which they then can afford to compress. These diagrams help to show the process we aim for in the groups.

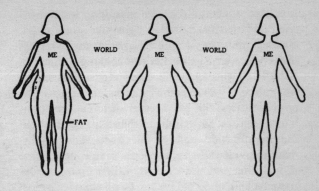

To help in the very difficult task of self-acceptance and the preparation for a new slim body and new self-image we employ the following strategies. Bear in mind that you first have to own something before you can lose it. You must first accept your body in its largeness before you can give it up. A full-length undistorted mirror is the first place to start. Group members set aside time each day—maybe just a couple of minutes at the outset—to observe their bodies. Most compulsive eaters are very aware of how their faces look but not in relation to the rest of their bodies. What we try to do in this exercise is to observe our bodies. We are using the mirror to see ourselves without judging the image it holds. This is both a frightening and difficult project for many women because one is so used to making a grimace and judgment on the few occasions we do see our whole bodies. We are so familiar with avoiding possibly unacceptable visions, keeping our heads down as we walk past shop windows lest we cast a glance at ourselves unaware and trigger negative feelings. So, in doing the exercise, a woman is asked initially to look at the reflected image of herself as she would a work of art, for example, a sculpture, getting to know its dimensions and texture. She is looking to find out where it begins and ends; where it curves or bumps in and out; what color changes there are. The woman tries this in several different positions starting first by standing, then sitting—without having to hide half of her body—and finally, standing sideways. Some people have a greater ease doing this exercise dressed; others find it more manageable nude. So we start with what feels most comfortable and stay with that until the woman can have the experience of looking in the mirror and not flashing to feelings of disgust.

The second step in the mirror exercise is aimed to help you experience yourself existing throughout your body. Many women experience their fat as something that surrounds them with their true selves inside or, alternatively, that their fat trails them, taking up more room than it really does. So when a woman is standing in front of the mirror the emphasis in this part of the exercise is to feel herself *throughout* her body. She follows her breath on its course from her lungs through her body. The large thighs she may wish to reject are as much a part of her body as the wrist that seems so much more acceptable. Try to see the various parts of your body as connected. Start with your toes and remind yourself of how your toes are connected to your feet and your feet are connected to your ankles and your ankles are connected to your lower leg, and so on. It will provide you with a holistic view of your body. You will begin to experience yourself as existing through the fat.

This new approach has another function. If you can experience yourself as existing throughout the fat, then when you lose weight, you will not feel you have lost a protective covering; you will feel you have become compressed. This is because if you feel yourself all through the fat then what is all of you is part of you. In giving up the size you are making an exchange—you swap the fat for your own body, and that is power.

The drawings are worth repeating here because these will help toward an understanding of what we are trying to achieve in reducing the discrepancy between the fat self and the small interior physical self. We are aiming for a situation where the sequence, me:fat:world, is replaced by me:world.

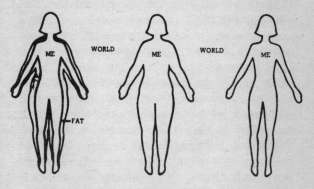

As I mentioned above, women report that when they have lost weight they have allowed themselves to wear very different clothes from those they wore when they considered their bodies as unacceptably large. A compulsive eater may have at least three wardrobes. These generally consist of one or two smocky-type items that will cover her at her absolute maximum weight; nondescript clothes for

a medium weight; and clothes for when she was or
will be thin which tend to be more stylish and varied
and allow for a greater range of expression. The
clothes in the larger sizes will almost undoubtedly
be circumscribed by what is available in the shops
and by what a compulsive eater thinks is permissible
to wear. When you look at the clothing racks in sizes
18, 20 and up there is much less variety and styling
than in the 10s and 12s. The taboos in people's
minds against bright colors, horizontal strips and
good design for fat people correspond to what is
available in the stores. By and large, cheap, stylish
clothing is not available over size 14. It is therefore
not surprising that when a woman loses weight she
can experiment with projecting different images
through her dressing, because for the first time
alternative clothing is readily available. However, it
is also true that as long as she feels her body size is
unacceptable, she will be using her clothing to hide
her body and avoid drawing attention to it. The
initial goal of the groups is to give each woman a
greater acceptance of her body. Without such
acceptance we maintain that weight loss will be
temporary because it will continue to trigger off
frightening feelings. To avoid this state we do
preparatory work in the area of body size, body
image and dressing. We encourage the women to
throw out or pack away or trade with other group
members, all the clothes in their closets that do not
currently fit them. This means that every morning,
instead of confronting three sets of clothes (indeed,
three different people in their closets) and torturing
themselves about the "thin" clothes that continually
await and attack them, they will be looking at the
clothes that do fit. Much of the compulsive eater's
negative self-image gets expressed in the way she

dresses and carries herself. This then produces a spiralling of self-hate. One woman I worked with said, "I feel ashamed of my body and I just cover it as efficiently as possible in a big smock. Then I realize I don't like my clothes either, so I end up doubly hating myself." Almost inevitably, these self-rejecting feelings lead the compulsive eater to cram food into her mouth to assuage the feelings and then, of course, come renewed recriminations and resolutions to start yet another diet.

Having bared one's wardrobe, we are ready to move to step two. This involves experimenting with various images of yourself and dressing to express those now, not waiting until you are thin to wear the kinds of clothes in which you imagine yourself thin. It is not a criminal act to tuck in your blouse, shirt or sweater when overweight. It rarely makes you look larger to be more defined. This latter idea is one of the misconceptions we carry around supposing that loose clothing makes us look less big than fitted clothing. It may attract more attention. If so, that gives you the opportunity to work on reactions to one of the imagined consequences of being thin. Better to test it out and see how it feels while you still have the safety of the fat. It is important to test out your ideas of the images you want to express to find out what really feels good and what feels scary. In the groups, women can get some feedback for the images they are projecting; they can discuss whether there is a discrepancy between what they wish to project and are indeed projecting. Group members can also help each other go shopping for clothes or material to make garments[1] and help each other through a day of real or imagined critical sales staff and fellow shoppers.

Mirror work and dressing for now are thus two

of the basic techniques used in the group to help women both accept their current body size and prepare for a smaller one. In addition, we encourage group members to adopt a self-image close to the one they imagine they will have when thin. This has its physical aspects as well as emotional ones, and an aim of the group is to work on the different levels simultaneously.

Another of the preparatory exercises employed is to imagine not only what you intend to project when thin through your clothing but also through body position and stance as well. Many women report that when they were thin before, they sat, stood and danced quite differently, generally adopting more open postures. These different stances produced a variety of effects, some of which they were comfortable with and others with which they were not. The difficult ones mainly had to do with others' responses and the women found that they did not know how to deal with people's reactions. Putting on weight again had been their only option. An illustration from my work with Janet describes well her actual experience of becoming thin in the past.

Janet is a twenty-six-year-old social worker in a drug-addiction agency. She grew up in Brooklyn, the eldest of three children in a middle-class Jewish family. She was of average weight until she was thirteen. Her mother was slightly overweight and from time to time was preoccupied with dieting. At the dinner table her mother would often be eating a modified version of the family meal—no potatoes or desserts. When Janet's body started to develop into that of a woman she put on about fifteen pounds. She felt quie uncomfortable with the changes going on in her body and she sought advice from the adolescent girls' magazines on how to cope with this new shape and the distressing feelings that accompanied puberty. She gravitated toward articles entitled, "How to Look Like a Happy Teenager; What to do about the changes going on in your body." Under cosy headlines these articles contained a ghastly message. Janet learned there was something decidedly wrong about her shape and was told that the answer lay in weight control. Thus started thirteen years of dieting and bingeing. Janet's initial experience of terror and anxiety about her body changes found no outlet except in these magazines. She had no other place to explore the revulsion, excitement and fear that she was feeling about periods, bras and pubic hair. Indeed, her introduction to her menstrual periods itself was quite confusing. Although prepared for the event so that she was not initially frightened when the blood began, she had no real way to understand the response from her mother. On telling her, she was slapped on the cheek[2] and offered congratulations. Subsequently, she overheard her mother telephoning family friends to announce with pride that Janet was a woman. Thus, an introduction to womanhood was accompanied by an act of violence. It was hard for Janet to put together the slap and the congratulations. The idea that she had done something wrong, or indeed was all wrong, provided the basis for her to latch on to those articles and advertisements which promised solutions to one's failures through attaining the correct body size. The very first diet she went on made her feel wonderful. She experienced it as an act of independence from her family. She would decide what to eat rather than eat whatever was put on the

table. The diet had a double edged function. She
could try and transform her body and she could
establish her separateness from the family. She
performed adequately academically and went away
to college and graduate school. When I first met
Janet she had been working for two years, she had a
large circle of friends which included some close
women friends, and had been living with Alan, an
architect, for over two years. With one exception,
she felt quite pleased with the way her life was going,
feeling herself to be quite active, social and
competent on the job. The one exception was her
obsession with weight, dieting and body size. She
was 5 feet 2 inches and felt overweight at 130
pounds. She had successfully dieted many times to
112 pounds but had never maintained the weight
loss for more than a few months. Her current weight
was not far off the maximum she had ever been. In
the course of the therapy we traced the different
times when her weight had increased and decreased.
As I have sketched out above we discussed in detail
the original feelings that had propelled her toward
the diet-binge syndrome. Two important discov-
eries were made. The first was that many times Janet
had geared up to diet and, having lost the weight,
felt herself attractive enough to get sexually
involved with men. These relationships varied in
length but almost inevitably her eating went
through three phases when she was sexually
involved. The first phase, which lasted a week or so,
was characterized by a startling lack of interest in
food. These were the only times since she was
thirteen that Janet can remember actually not being
preoccupied with her food intake. She ate quite little
and was not particularly aware of how it tasted. The

length of the second phase varied. With Alan she kept quite close to her diet for about three months, with no significant weight variation but with a considerable preoccupation and worry about food with days defined as "good" or "bad"—depending on her intake. After three months they went on vacation together and Janet relaxed the proscription on her consumption of food although her obsession was just as great. Privately, she judged, worried or praised herself according to what passed between her lips. She resolved to diet when she got back from their vacation. Meanwhile, she ate a wide range of foods, particularly the kind of which she deprived herself during the previous months. When she and Alan returned to New York she had put on enough weight to convince herself that she must diet yet again. For the next fifteen months she yoyoed but became increasingly bored and unconvinced by the whole approach.

So one pattern was: weight loss to sexual involvement to weight gain. The other instances when she lost weight corresponded to big changes in her life—entry into high school, leaving home to go to college, leaving college and taking summer jobs, the beginning of the year she worked between college and graduate school and the return to New York City to work in the drug-addiction agency. Each one of these occasions represented Janet's growing independence and autonomy. She met them with confidence and a slim body and was quite perplexed as to why the impulse to eat compulsively returned shortly after she had settled in new surroundings.

In the course of the therapy, Janet described her experiences in sexual relationships and with new

places, jobs and school challenges. What began to
emerge was that the issues of separation and
sexuality were more difficult for her than she had
been aware of. In her sexual relationships she was
able to see that she believed her acceptance was
based on her looking a particular way and being
thin. She received plenty of sexual attention which,
although she enjoyed, threatened her—she did not
know how to turn people away. She also did not
know if she was as sexual inside as she projected
outside because, in her periods of weight gain, she
did not feel at all sexual and had not met with much
sexual interest from others. In addition, she worried
that she might become uncontrollably promiscuous
if she were thin all the time. Her mother's attitude
toward her was painful and confusing. Whereas her
mother had previously encouraged dieting, she now
passed comments on how Janet was looking pale
and as if she might disappear. Janet had not become
the thin, beautiful daughter her mother had wanted,
and she was hurt by her mother's ambivalence
toward her newfound self-acceptance. She was also
confused by the reactions of men; she could not
seem to please both her mother and men at the same
time.

As we replayed her feelings frame by frame,
Janet sensed the vulnerability she experienced in
herself as a thin woman. She felt that she had
become what everyone had encouraged her to be
and was met by disapproval from her mother on the
one hand, and abundant sexual interest from men
on the other. She realized that she felt quite unable
to handle these two kinds of attention. The
disapproval from her mother made no sense to her
and Janet felt angry as though she were being

betrayed. She felt quite inadequate to handle all the sexual attention and felt that she had no way to say "yes" or "no" in a way which corresponded to her own desires. She felt she had no tools by which to select whomever she was interested in but, perhaps more confusing, she felt that now she had a beautiful body she was required to project the sexuality she had hidden in her overweight periods.

In dealing with the theme of separation, Janet realized that as she had taken on the new challenges at school, college, and in her job, she had, indeed, been quite worried about what was expected of her. She had coped with her anxieties by attempting to take a hold of herself—putting herself on a stringent diet. When she started college she projected an image, and attempted to believe in that image of herself—one that expressed independence, competence, interest and general enthusiasm. Underneath this construct, and into the diet, were placed her fears of inadequacy, loneliness, boredom and lack of security. She rarely allowed herself to have those feelings for more than an instant and set herself the task of living up to her idealized self-image as a thin person.

As she realized how ungenerous she had been to herself in her thin times, so it emerged how much of an investment she had made in being thin whenever she put on weight. To be thin was a state that allowed no pain, no mistakes and represented independence and sexuality.

In the therapy we worked toward Janet's acknowledgment of just how scary her past experiences of being thin were. Having seen this, Janet looked to aspects of herself that she left behind in the fat. She began to incorporate those into an idea of herself thin. She learned how to be assertive so that she could say "yes" or "no" in sexual and other situations rather than being the victim of her body size. She looked at the feelings that seemed unacceptable while she was thin and began to articulate them directly rather than hiding them within the fat so that when she lost the weight again she was sure she could express them directly then and did not worry that she had no place to hide them. She allowed herself the possibility that she could be thin and have conflicts; that whatever conflicts she had with her mother, with her own sexuality, with her anger or whatever, they could all exist as part of her when thin. This did not mean resolving all the difficulties but acknowledging and accepting them. It meant giving up the idea that being thin meant that her life had to work out right all the time.

The actual progress of Janet's therapy was, of course, not a straightforward march with one theme unfolding after the other in the orderly fashion I described above. Insights and realizations come suddenly, fade away and come back again. Only through fantasy work, slow loss of weight, intermittent bingeing, and the hard work necessary to try out the insights in fearful situations, does such a complete picture emerge. Janet's therapy lasted fourteen months after which she had completely broken the compulsion and had lost weight. She stabilized at about 112–114 pounds. Follow-up sessions verified that the understanding Janet had reached about her own experience of eating had permitted her to remain permanently at the weight she desired. She had found more direct and assertive ways for dealing with the problems of sexuality and womanhood than body size.

For Janet then, work on the meanings of fat and thin provided her with the opportunity to change her self-image. She closed the gap between her fantasies of who she would be thin and who she was in reality. This exploration and then abandonment of the thin fantasies allowed her to give up unrealistic expectations of personality change.

As we have seen, women unconsciously fear being thin. If one is thin then one is expected to fit the norm. If one is thin others will equate comforming in body size with conforming with stereotyped female behavior. If one is thin, how can one be self-defining? It is precisely these confusions that have kept many women away from permanent thinness, and it is these underlying issues that need to be confronted so that a woman can experience the choice of being thin *and* herself.

It takes quite a bit of unraveling to separate the threads that push women to lose weight one week and gain it the next. In clarifying the tensions, I have tried to identify the varied reasons why thinness may be feared. A major question that needs to be confronted individually is, "How will I be who I wish to be if I look as I am supposed to look?" Consideration of this question is essential and goes a long way toward providing solutions to being a thin woman in this culture.

The experience of
hunger for the
compulsive eater

The women I see have already tried many different ways to lose weight including hypnosis, Weight Watchers Inc., diet doctors, cellulose fillers, appetite suppressants and diuretics, Overeaters Anonymous and magic. All these methods are external schemes. Food intake is limited and particular foods—such as ice cream, cake and bread—are banned. This is all based on the principle that if you reduce your caloric intake (or carbohydrate intake) you will lose weight. Diets range from Stillman's Water Diet to Atkin's and the Mayo Clinic Diet, from the Banana Diet to the Drinking Person's

Diet. A million diets and a million dieters. Millions of dollars too: ten billion dollars is spent annually by the American public to get thin and stay thin.[1]

All these diets and weight-reduction schemes have two things in common. First, there is a devastatingly high rate of recidivism. Dieters lose weight by the ton but their success in keeping their weight down is less formidable.[2] Statistics are scarce but the maintenance rates are rumored to be scandalously low. The second feature these schemes share is a stress on reinforcing the compulsive activity and an emphasis on cultural stereotypes of thinness and fatness.

None of these plans addresses the central issues behind compulsive eating. Two of these issues are the experience of hunger and the need to break food addiction. "Fat people" are not as aware of the actual mechanism of hunger as "normal weight" non-compulsive eaters.[3] This means that compulsive eaters do not use their gurgling stomachs to tell them when to eat. Eating becomes so loaded with other meanings that a straightforward reaction to a hungry stomach is unusual. Indeed one of the features of compulsive eating is eating in such a way that physical hunger is never felt. The social stigma attached to being overweight accentuates this problem. Fat people in our culture feel the stigma in this way; "Fat is bad, I should always be trying to lose weight and I definitely should not enjoy food." In general, compulsive eaters divide food into categories of "good foods" and "bad foods." All the diets work on the principle that food is dangerous. Only through rigorous deprivation can the compulsive eater redeem herself, lose weight and begin to enjoy life. So the mechanism of hunger on which "normal" eaters rely is distorted. Years of guilty eating and mammoth deprivation schemes mean that the compulsive eater is very out of touch with the experience of hunger and the ability to satisfy it.

Distortions of the eating process cause confusion for the compulsive eater while the myriad of weight-reduction schemes infantilize her and reduce her control over her own eating to a minimum. As anyone who has ever dieted knows, the structure of a diet is rigid. Diets become moral straitjackets which confine the compulsive eater. *In turning to dieting, all the compulsiveness evident in overeating is now channeled into a new obsession—to staying on the diet.* Follow these rules, eat what the authorities tell you. Above all, do what women are so good at—deprive yourself. Even the so-called liberal diets ("Eat fat and grow slim," "Enjoy as much food and vegetables as you like") rely on a structure that disenfranchizes the woman from her own body. "Eat bananas seven times a day; weigh four ounces of fish and three ounces of grated cheese; drink one glass of pulp-free orange juice a day and unlimited cups of black coffee or tea; use one bowl only and eat with chopsticks; always eat in the same place or at the same time; always eat a big breakfast; eat starch, cut out fat; cut out fat but eat high protein; lose weight and *get/hold your man.*" But never, never let yourself go or find out what you like to eat, when or how.

In the main, the compulsive eater knows two realities: compulsive eating (out of control) or compulsive dieting (imprisonment). To be a compulsive eater means to be a food junkie. Compulsive eaters crave their food as badly as a junkie craves heroin or an alcoholic thirsts for liquor. They spend much of their energy battling against their addiction. They are always going "cold turkey"—dieting or fasting—or trying their methadone substitute—cottage cheese. While a drug addict or alcoholic is not continually struggling against the heroin or liquor, the compulsive eater is caught in an antagonistic relationship with the food she so wants. While the junkie may spend hours hustling the money and connection for the next fix, the compulsive eater will devote the same kind of psychic energy working out what to eat or not. In the end, as the heroin "fixes" the drug addict and the liquor "stuporizes" the alcoholic, so the binge "narcotizes" the compulsive eater.

A curious aspect in the compulsive eater's addiction is that from a look at her kitchen or her public eating one might get the impression that certain foods are illegal. The presence of particular foods is so rare, and ingestion so clandestine, that one might be forgiven for assuming that criminal penalties are given for the possession and consumption of certain foods. It is as though foods are classified, with ice-cream sundaes and French fries as felonies; bananas and cream as misdemeanors and food in general as a violation. In fact, one well-known slimming organization characterizes food in just this way. Some foods are legal and can be eaten incessantly and in unlimited quantities, others are illegal and are to be eaten only in a restricted way. Thus the compulsive eater is encouraged to create her own jail sentence and in doing so she faces the world very much as does the junkie or alcoholic. This tension converts food into an enemy or an evil to be warded off constantly while at the same time it provides, however shortlived, a treat and comfort.

Unlike other addicts, however, the compulsive eater can find temporary relief in not eating. Not eating means she is being "good" and conjures up immediate images of the rewards to come from thinness. Contrary to popular images of greed, the compulsive eater is quite frightened of food and what it can do to her. Short spells of withdrawal remove her from the responsibility of what she is putting in her mouth. The food is a drug, it is magical, it is poison, it is to keep one alive, it is suffocating, it is tantalizing, but only very rarely is it seen as an essential enjoyable aspect of life. It is from this fear of food that the compulsive eater's large appetite springs. The compulsive eater can eat a lot of food. Often she does not taste the three boxes of cookies, ten celery stalks, four packets of potato chips and frozen pizza that she can consume at one sitting. The food is so guiltily eaten that enjoyment is limited. The feeling of insatiability is very strong and the compulsive eater will cram seemingly unappetizing foods, like dry cereal, into her mouth during a binge. The food must be eaten quickly so that it is no longer dangerous. Once consumed, the crisis has passed and the compulsive eater is left with the familiar bad feelings following a binge.

Compulsive eating means eating without regard to the physiological cues which signal hunger. People who have never had difficulty distinguishing hunger pangs take it for granted that their bodies are wanting food then. They may be quite astonished by the extent to which this mechanism is so underutilized by the compulsive eater. For a compulsive eater it is an equally astonishing idea that people who do not have difficulty with food rely on their stomachs to tell them what, how much and when to eat. For the compulsive eater, food has taken on such additional significance that it has long since lost its obvious biological connection.

The word "hunger" usually connotes the desire to eat. The body is depleted and needs nourishment. In its extreme form hunger becomes starvation. In its current Western setting the satisfaction of hunger is a social experience. While there is controversy about what exactly constitutes hunger, and what controls appetite and satisfaction, it is strikingly clear that the compulsive eater very rarely eats in response to the stomach cues which signal hunger.[4] Indeed, when we introduce this possibility as an important way out of the whole syndrome, people are eager to be reintroduced to aspects of their bodies they have ignored for so long. While one is rejecting one's body, an enormous alienation exists between it and oneself. This estrangement makes it hard to be receptive to signals from the body. If you have never felt your body was alright or acceptable but was cumbersome, unattractive or not pleasing in some way, it is quite a leap to trust what it has to say, as if an enemy territory were commanding. To listen to a body that has constantly been an unseemly colony is to own that body. To own your own body means to take its needs seriously and disregard many of the external values and measures to which you have attempted to mold it. This distortion of the hunger mechanism does not have a clear origin and it may begin very early on in life. What is clear is that many young women begin to tamper with this mechanism in an effort to transform their bodies at the time of puberty. An analogy may make this distortion process more graphic for those who have considerable difficulty envisaging hunger and an appropriate response. Take, for example, a tickle in the throat. This feeling is satisfied by a cough. A sneeze is preceded by a slight irritation in the nostrils. These reactions are virtually involuntary and few people suffer from the continual need to deny a cough or a sneeze, on the odd occasion it may be polite to stifle the sneeze or cough but not on a continuing basis.

Another example in which one acts less automatically is when one's bladder is full and there is a need to release the pressure. Again, most people will grow up with a confidence about knowing how to follow the signals that they need to urinate and the amount will vary considerably. Sometimes there will be a great deal of pressure on the bladder, sometimes less, but the information that one needs relief will become available quite obviously. These three physical activities are all under self-regulation and depend for satisfaction on recognition of the cues. This is true for the hunger mechanism too. The infant has the capacity to develop a harmonious relationship with its various bodily needs. It can learn to identify hunger cues and feel contented when satisfactorily fed. The confidence that there will be satisfaction is shaped by positive interaction with the environment. When a child cries from hunger and is fed, and cries for affection and gets held, then her cues will have been responded to appropriately and as the child develops she will be able to trust that she can both recognize and fulfill her needs.

Many women who have compulsive-eating problems do not feel confident that they can recognize their signs of hunger and then eat to fulfill them. Not only has the hunger process been abused through years of dieting and bingeing but pre-puberty eating is often remembered as tortured, interrupted and conflicted. In tracing back, we surmise that such a woman's very early signs of bodily needs were misinterpreted by her mother so that there is confusion over a variety of physical sensations. For example, it every time a child cries it is answered with food, then the food takes on the role of comforter. However, if a baby's diaper needs changing or a baby wants some kind of physical contact, providing food will give neither satisfaction or comfort, nor will it allow the infant to develop trust in its own body. Feeding in response to other bodily needs alienates a child from its body and interferes with the individual's ability to recognize both hunger and satisfaction. This early distortion may well be a contributing factor to many women's discomfort with their own bodies; a discomfort which is then readily available to manipulation by how society says one *should* look and what one *should* eat. Outside cues become powerful sources on which to rely in the absence of confidence that one can take care of one's own needs. Diet sheets and bakeries are equal contenders when a woman is seeking information about how to care for herself. Often compulsive eaters will describe their current eating in a way that confirms our impression that early satisfaction was interfered with. Daphne, a thirty-two-year-old librarian, described much of her eating as a search for something that is missing. "When I go to the refrigerator I'm quite aware that it is not food I am actually after but it's as though I'm looking for a missing piece." The missing piece turns out to be a general unease and unsureness about whether she can provide adequately for her own needs.

This discourse on hunger and the distortion of the mechanism is not meant to put the blame on mothers for misinterpreting their children's body signals. It is true that in their role as primary caretakers, they often do misinterpret their infants' needs, but an explanation that stops there misses crucial issues that affect all women. The question is more *why* mothers give their children food when that is not what they may be wanting. Why is it that food is always at the ready to be offered when the child expresses discomfort? What are the social forces that produce this kind of mothering? We look for the answer in the social position of women. It is in her role as mother that a woman is unequivocally accepted. It is in her role as mother that she is counseled to be attentive and nurturing to her child. Nearly all of us will have grown up at a time when child care was seen to be the province of mothers. They were seen as the only ones who could adequately care for their children and establish the emotional bonding considered crucial for "healthy" development. However, while considered the essential figure in the infant's daily life, the mother is not considered expert on child rearing. Instead, she will be encouraged to draw on the expertise of a wide range of specialists—pediatricians, child psychologists, analysts, nutritionists—who will tell her how, when and what she should or should not feed her child. Most "experts" contradict each other as the fashion in child rearing changes and the different disciplines rush to fit their theories into prevailing ideologies.

Thus the mother is acclaimed on the one hand as *the* only suitable primary caretaker but on the other, is considered to be inadequately prepared to cope with this job and must rely on conflicting "expert" opinions. If is in this situation that the woman comes to motherhood and the care of her child, and it is not surprising that she then distrusts her own reactions to her child's signals. Alternately deified and devalued, it is hard for her to feel secure about her own responses. One can well imagine how this insecurity is readily reinforced by other consequences of an enforced maternal role. As a mother, this is the chance in life to have an impact on shaping an aspect of one's world (through the child). This may set off in the mother feelings of delight, inadequacy, fear, insecurity, resentment or enthusiasm which are then expressed through her contact with the child. A mother's fears of inadequacy may cause her to overfeed her child by feeding it automatically every time it cries, just as her resentment at being its sole nurse may make her neglect it. But another factor may be involved: when a child cries and expresses its distress and, as the mother imagines, helplessness, she may see herself as the parent who must respond but also, find her own painful feelings of early deprivation reevoked. If *we* are "inadequate mothers," we are also daughters of "inadequate mothers" who were themselves daughters. If the early distortion in the feeding relationship is attributable to the social forces present in the mother-daughter relationship, then this will be as true for our mothers as daughters, and our mother's mothers as daughters. As long as a patriarchal culture demands that women bring up their daughters to accept an inferior social position, the mother's job will be fraught with tension and confusion which are often made manifest in the way mothers and daughters interact over the subject of food.

The experience of hunger, then, will not be the compulsive eater's motive for eating. She will not experience her eating as self-regulatory but as a kind of outside force tempting, pleasing and betraying her. Once overweight she will most probably adopt an attitude that says she is not entitled to eat, as though fatness can only be excused, or as if fat people only have a right to exist if they do not eat. Fat people move into a category quite apart from the rest of the population. While advertisers court us to eat more and more, slimming columns, doctors, fashion magazines and friends counsel those overweight to curtail their food intake. But to tell a compulsive eater to control something she feels is out of her control has the effect of making her feel powerless and guilty; powerless for being so apparently ineffectual and guilty for whatever food she does eat. This guilt further distances her from discovering what it is she would *like* to eat because she has become preoccupied with what she *should* or *should not* eat. Food is something to be feared, and to eat feels like committing a sin, for one feels so undeserving and unentitled. Eating takes place quickly and frequently furtively.

A compulsive eater would describe this experience in one of several ways:

1. FOOD AS SOCIAL: "I'm never hungry at suppertime but I like everyone to eat together because it *feels*

like we are a happy family if we eat together.
Mealtimes are significant not for the food but for
the appearance of family closeness."

2. MOUTH HUNGER: "I really need to put some food
in my mouth although I don't feel hungry in my
stomach."

3. EATING PROPHYLACTICALLY: "I'm not hungry at
the moment but I might be hungry in a couple of
hours and I won't be able to get anything then, so I'd
better have some food now."

4. DESERVED FOOD: "I had a ghastly day. I think I'll
cheer myself up with a nice nosh."

5. GUARANTEED PLEASURE: "Eating goodies is the
only way to give myself a real treat. It's the one
pleasure that I know how to give myself."

6. NERVOUS EATING: "I just have to have something.
What can I cram into my mouth?"

7. CELEBRATORY EATING: "I had such a great day,
one packet of Fritos can't possibly hurt me."

8. EATING OUT OF BOREDOM: "I'm not in the mood to
do anything at the moment ... I'll fix myself a club
sandwich."

With compulsive dieting there is *also* no response
to physiological hunger. The dieter is eating out of a
prescribed set of rules saying what foods are allowed
or forbidden; she is eating at specified mealtimes
with little regard for what her body wants and when
it wants it.

We work on the premise that compulsive eaters

*do not really allow themselves to eat, and conse-
quently are either stuffing their mouths or depriving
themselves. Every time a compulsive eater goes on a
diet she is telling herself that there is something
wrong with her so she must deprive herself.* She
defines her current self as reprehensible, so she
decides to punish herself through denial. In this
way, the compulsive eater rarely allows herself the
direct pleasure that food can bring. A vicious circle
ensues. While she may eat everything in sight when
she is not dieting for fear of imminent deprivation,
she is nevertheless not enjoying the food. "I ate
twenty cookies in ten minutes today. Tomorrow I'm
going to put myself on a diet during which I won't be
able to have any cookies, so I had to get all my
cookie eating in today before I have to be good." At
the same time the twenty cookies are also a rebellion
against the non-entitlement and deprivation.

This diet-binge syndrome can be broken by the
compulsive eater when she begins to see herself as a
"normal" person, with fat being nothing more than
a descriptive word, without connoting good or bad.
If the compulsive eater can begin to experience
herself as "normal" then she can begin to eat like a
"normal" person. This means learning to recognize
the difference between real hunger and psychological hunger, and eating accordingly. It means eating
enough to satisfy one's hunger and eating whatever
food satisfies that particular hunger (be it donuts or
steak). After all, people without a compulsive-
eating problem do not deprive themselves of food
by choice. In observing the eating behavior of
people who do not suffer over food, it is interesting
to note just what a wide range of foods they do eat
and how much at variance with conceptions of

"healthy diet" their daily intake may be. It is also important to realize that they occasionally overeat for pleasure. As this eating is not a substitute for other needs it does not have other connotations. It is the driving compulsion to stuff or starve that we are trying to dissolve rather than dictating "correct" amounts of food intake.

To find out what, when and how much you might like to eat is not as simple as it seems. In addition, the pressure of the diet and fashion industry, which spends incalculable amounts of money making sure that women do not themselves decide what they would like to eat and wear, reinforces the idea that the compulsive eater is irresponsible, out of control, negligent and hateful.

On the psychological level the experience of hunger pangs can be quite scary. Some of the fear comes from an anxiety about one's ability to satisfy bodily hunger: "If I'm not stuffing my face or starving myself, what should I do? How will I know how much to eat? Maybe I'll never want to stop."

Another frightening factor is related to a challenge of the "female-as-child" concept. For if you can respond to the hunger cues that your body does indeed transmit, this places you in a situation where you might actually satisfy yourself and begin to be in harmony with your body. This idea of being able to take care of yourself allows you to see the female as an adult with the rights and privileges that other adults (male adults) have. This means taking your own needs seriously and attempting to satisfy them for yourself. A woman is brought up to be attuned to and satisfy others' needs. The struggle to know what you want or need to eat changes the way you respond to others' needs. As you begin to trust the capacity to feed yourself you find a basis for being more explicit in relation to other needs. "If I can take care of myself with food and say 'yes' and 'no' to what I am wanting or not wanting, then I can spell out for myself, *and* to others, desires in other areas and feel more in charge of other aspects of my life." Being able to act on one's own needs is a novel experience and one overwhelmingly denied to women in this culture.

When the compulsive eater imagines herself as a thin female adult, when everything else in her life is supposed to hang together better, she has to conform to an image of womanhood rather than be confident with who she is. While this idea is fantasy, it is nevertheless a powerful and scary one: "If I am thin, and look like a 'real' woman, then I must be productive, energetic, together and loving." The struggle to be female and self-defined is hard, with few supports for an expression of true female personhood.

In our work we spend a great deal of time uncovering and demystifying the various fantasies associated with fat and thin. At the same time we work together on the technical side, learning new ways to approach food and hunger. The steps that I outline here start with the idea that we are not going to judge whatever it is that we eat. Rather, we are going to observe the ways in which we eat. Learning not to judge one's food intake is not very easy. Years of attempting to follow the rules do not quickly fade away. To observe an aspect of the self which has been rejected time and time again requires a good deal of self-acceptance. Turning off one's judges— mothers, women's magazines, husbands, lovers, friends, diet doctors and nutritionists—requires trust in one's self. Being in a group with other women going through the same process can be of great assistance and support.

The first step is to learn about your eating patterns. This means pinpointing those times when you feel particularly vulnerable to attack by the food and to notice any occasions when you feel more at ease with it. By noting your food intake for a short period you will both gather data and develop a sense of yourself as an observer. As an observer you can begin to see that there is a part of you that eats and another part that does other things, including being an observer. Then you have broken away from the idea of yourself as being someone who is obsessed with food. You are ready to move on to becoming a "normal" person who eats like "normal" people.

Now the second step is taken. We move from observation to action. First, we begin to identify the difference between mouth hunger and stomach hunger. Risk going without food for a couple of waking hours until you experience some hunger sensations in your body. Most probably you will feel it in your stomach, though some people feel it in the chest or throat. When you feel the difference between the two types of hunger, see how it feels for a minute or so. Is it reassuring or scary? Do you associate pleasant or unpleasant memories with it? Often the first realized feelings of stomach hunger may produce painful associations which you will want to examine with your group or on your own. Mimi, a woman we worked with, discovered that when she allowed herself to experience hunger pangs, she got in touch with a whole other range of body emotions that she had successfully been trying to hide from herself. She felt sexual. These sexual feelings made her quite uncomfortable because she had come to think of sexuality as sinful, or not appropriate for herself. In talking about what this meant she was able to separate hunger pangs from guilt-producing sexuality. Another woman, Betty, remembered being hungry as a child when there was not enough food on the table. And Martha, whose family urged her to eat, discovered for herself that hungry feelings expressed capitulation to the family feeding situation. The process of working through these particular situations was enriched by a feminist understanding of the particular problems they each expressed. For instance, in examining Mimi's response to her sexual feelings we explored why and how she learned that sex was sinful for her, for women. In exploring Betty's hunger as a child we brought into focus the painful lot of mothers who hold back when there is not enough food and encourage the children to eat. Betty discovered that she actually denied herself more than necessary in an identification with her mother at the family table. To be a woman meant to be self-denying. Martha's giving in at the table reflected for her an ambivalence in separating from her family, a difficulty particularly acute for women where separation has traditionally occurred only at marriage. Looking at these associations in these ways can provide useful clues to the roots of your own particular history with food. Ultimately, when you have learned to give your body exactly what it wants you will be able to look forward to those hunger pangs because it is a message that your body is wanting something delicious.

The next step is to eat out of stomach hunger

only as much as possible. Do not worry too much about this at first, because anyone with a history of compulsive eating is bound occasionally to eat from mouth hunger. But try to begin to see your body as a finely tuned instrument that likes to be lovingly cared for. When it is very hungry it might want quite a bit of nourishment; when it is only mildly hungry, quite a little less. In line with this, having learned about stomach hunger, try to locate precisely what food or liquid your body is hungry for. That is, once having experienced hunger pangs, work out what particular food or foods will satisfy that particular hunger. Sometimes this will be very easy and you will know right away what it is you are wanting, but often, particularly because of the years of "shoulds" and regimens, you might not know and in this case you might find a two-minute fantasy exercise helpful. Close your eyes and ask yourself "What kind of physical sensation do I have and how can I best satisfy it? Do I want something crunchy, salty, chewy, moist, sweet? Okay, I want some potato chips. Let me imagine myself eating some. No, that's not it. How about some plain chocolate...?"

In this way before you eat the food you will have already imagined how it is most likely going to feel going down. Taste the soup traveling down your throat, bite on the nuts, smell the fresh bread in your fantasy. Find the foods that fit the mood and then eat. Eat as much as your body is wanting. Really taste each mouthful. Enjoy yourself.

Quite frequently, no food will clearly present itself and this can mean one of two things. You are hungry but cannot find exactly what would make sense. Have a little of a food you enjoy and wait till you get a clear message. You may have let the hunger go on too long so that your stomach is jumping up and down and does not know how to be soothed. Alternatively you may not be hungry for food and it will be important for you to "feed" yourself more appropriately with a hug, a cry, a bath, a telephone conversation or a run. If it *is* something else you are wanting, food will not satisfy the original desire. At the very most, it can provide a temporary relief from feelings that creep up. What is more disturbing is that eating at these times serves to mask other urges and distances you further from the capacity to take care of yourself. Sort out what emotional need you are asking the food to carry for you and ask yourself whether indeed it works. As you discover how unsatisfactory this way of operating is, consider alternative ways to cope with your needs. If you are accustomed to eating compulsively during especially upsetting times, it will be reassuring to know you can feed yourself according to hunger and leave space to feel the distress. As Carol Bloom puts it in her training manual,[5] "Most compulsive eaters increase their non-nurturing eating during stress which usually makes them feel a lot worse. To not eat during those times (when you don't want to) is once again reinforcing a message to yourself, 'I can take care of myself, I can give myself the support I need.' 'It's a way not to desert yourself when things get tough.'"

For many people particular foods have special significance and correlate with particular moods and memories. Some like the calming effects of soup when they are feeling tense, carrots when they are angry or juice when they are feeling energetic. While I am not suggesting that you bite away your anger into a carrot and do not express it elsewhere, nevertheless food can be expressive. The main point is to pamper yourself with food—to allow every eating experience to be a pleasurable one—to see your stomach hunger as a signal for you to enjoy. Do not worry about regulation mealtimes or balanced meals. We do not believe in good foods or bad foods. *We believe that our bodies can tell us what to eat, how to have a nutritionally balanced food intake and how to lose weight.* The body is a self-regulatory system if allowed to operate. We are not concerned with caloric or carbohydrate value. Take a multivitamin pill every day until you feel that your body is as self-regulating as we propose it can be.

Now these suggestions—eat when you are hungry, eating as much as you want—may sound like a new set of rules that you are supposed to follow. In a sense they are. But we see them rather as helpful guidelines designed to let you trust your own bodily processes and as such, will not be experienced as "shoulds" but as guides until you experience total trust. In a sense, the steps outlined above are no more than a frame-by-frame description of what goes on for "normal" eaters.

Attention to the details of eating is a first step toward having a "normal" relationship with food. As you can say "yes" to a particular food so the possibility is there for you to say "no" to particular foods at particular times. Saying "no" is a great tool in self-definition but it is predicated on the ability to be able to say "yes" in a wholesome, guilt-free way.

A few more tips in demystifying food may be helpful. Try leaving a mouthful of every kind of food and drink you are ingesting on your plate, cup or glass. This will have two functions. On the one hand, it will begin to put the food at your control and reduce the feeling of insatiability; on the other, it will allow you to reject food. As you get more comfortable you will be able to define precisely how much food you are wanting. This exercise helped Elizabeth, a thirty-eight-year-old mother of three, who was brought up in England during the Second World War. It broke through a pattern she had established years back in trying to leave food on her plate. She had an image of her mother standing over her telling her she must not leave a crumb because soldiers had risked their lives getting the food to her. Food was rationed and goodies infrequent and Elizabeth felt she did not know when she would eat again.

Try loading up your house with "bad foods" that you feel attracted to and scared of. One woman we worked with was persuaded to keep enough ingredients for seventy-five ice-cream sundaes with all the trimmings. When it was first suggested that she fill the refrigerator with ice cream, sauce, nuts and cream she exclaimed, "But I'll eat it all!" The idea seemed so sinful to her. It was pointed out that if she had enough supplies for a minor army and could prove to herself that she did not want to consume it all at once, she would feel much more powerful and more in control of her food. She learned to love the ice cream and treat it as a friend to be called on when she wanted it rather than as an enemy to be conquered. She also took special care always to have plenty of her favorite brand or flavor. If you are really wanting to have coffee ice cream, the chocolate fudge in your refrigerator is a mediocre substitute. *It is worth going out to buy exactly what you want rather than just eating anything that is around.*

The only restrictions on this scheme are economic. It is unfortunate to have a yearning for fine smoked salmon when your pocketbook can only afford something cheaper. But really think about it. How much money did you used to spend on diet foods, diet books and binges?

In the groups we play a game to help focus on particular foods, and to destroy the idea that it is dangerous to have delicious foods in the house. We imagine that we have a special room filled with all of our favorite foods, and we see what it would be like to be surrounded with all of these wonderful taste possibilities. In the fantasy we see how it feels. Is it reassuring or scary to have all this goodness at one's fingertips? For most people it turns out that the initial flash makes them nervous. "I'll never get out the door! I'll always be eating!" But then, sitting with the fantasy for a minute or two, we find that people feel safe and protected with all the food around. They even find they have other things to do apart from preparing and eating food. If the food is there, if they know that they are never again going to deprive themselves by their own hands, then they can begin to get on with the business of living, and to start to eat in order to live rather than living in order to eat.

All the work you do on locating your hunger and learning how to satisfy it can be accompanied by an examination of the psychological issues that interfere with your ability to satisfy your food needs. For example, if you experience difficulty in allowing yourself to feel hunger, pay attention to both the physical sensations in the body as well as the psychological factors that prevent you from hearing what your body might be wanting. The psychological issues might range from doubts about your ability to nurture yourself and what it would mean to nurture yourself, to whose power you might be jeopardizing if you were to give to yourself. One woman discovered that, as she began to take her own needs seriously and specifically, she called into question her role in her family which was to take care of everybody else's needs while ignoring her own. Putting herself first in the food department was initially problematic for her. She felt she would be deserting her children. She found out subsequently that as she allowed herself to eat what she wanted, the whole family became more autonomous in that area. Mealtimes became much less tense affairs. Each member of the family chipped in to make something they wanted, and although there was some chaos while everyone was experimenting and messing up the kitchen, in the end each family member determined more of her or his own food intake and, as it turned out, took more responsibility in other areas of household labor.

Some people will find that as they begin to feel less addicted to food in general, certain foods will continue to have "magical" qualities. One woman I was seeing inexplicably ate candy periodically during the day while she was at work. We discovered that the intake of sweets had to do with the attempt to sweeten herself, to make herself "nice" when indeed she was feeling quite angry but felt that, "Women shouldn't get mad; it's not nice. I'd better make myself like sweet and spice." It turned out that she felt angry every time her boss

treated her in a way that was particularly demean-
ing. Although she was paid to do research she was
also expected to "serve." She was expected to
prepare the coffee and entertain the various male
clients that came to her office. These expectations
were examples of the sexual inequality that so often
operates in offices, and she, like many other women,
experienced conflict and rage when "feminized" in
such a way. In the group we role-played ways for her
to be more assertive with her boss and to discuss
with him other options for the preparation of coffee.
When a more equitable work situation was arrived
at she found less need to cram her mouth furtively
with candies. That is not to say that all her anger
disappeared. There are bound to be frictions as long
as there are bosses, but the anger was acknowledged
and validated by the group for what it was and
became separated from her eating activity.

In all that I have said it is important to remember
that our goal is not primarily weight loss. *The goal is
for the compulsive eater to break her addictive
relationship toward food.* While weight loss is
generally an important sign that the addiction is
broken, our primary concern is that you begin to
feel more comfortable about food. This cannot be
stressed too strongly. *The problem that we seek to
solve is addiction to food.* Continued obsession with
weight loss or gain hinders the process of learning to
love food and eating what your body is wanting.
While this process is not a magical shortcut, its
philosophy provides a basis for a more natural and
relaxed relationship toward food, and our bodies.

Self-help

If you see yourself as a compulsive eater the chances are that you know other women in the same position. Indeed, it is likely that you have dieted, fasted or gorged with friends even though the compulsive eating may be experienced as a solitary and even masturbatory activity. Women with a compulsive-eating problem tend to seek out others who will be sympathetic and understanding and it is largely true that the only people who can be really so are those who suffer from the same problem. If you do not feel close to anyone who shares this problem you can put up a notice in your college, community

center or women's center, in order to contact others
who might be interested in a self-help group. If you
feel reluctant to work in a group, the exercises
discussed can easily be done on your own. I do,
however, suggest that you consider working in a
group for the reasons I detail below.

There are several reasons for working on this
issue in a group. Some are practical and others are
related to the nature of the problem itself. On the
practical level there are not enough people doing
this work to satisfy the demand and interest for
individual therapy dealing with compulsive eating.
As more people who have had the problem and gone
through it, train and initiate work with others there
will be more options for those people who prefer
one-to-one settings. But for now I should like to
outline the advantages of group work and suggest a
model for a self-help group.

For those who have not had friendships solidi-
fied on the basis of sharing eating obsessions,
coming together with others who have the same
problem can be an enormous relief. To be able to
meet and talk with other women about this issue can
help relieve those terrible feelings of being an
isolated freak and a failure. Even for women who
have talked endlessly about food obsessions with
friends, the previous chats may have been circumscribed by the strictures of talking about diets
or diet foods. Grouping with other women to
explore explicitly one's relationship to fat and thin
can provide a comforting and safe experience. *For
some women it is like coming out of the closet. This
may be particularly the case for those women who
have managed to keep their weight within the
cultural norm so that nobody else is aware of their*

problem. For others, it is the relief of a supportive environment in which there is space for the grief and pain associated with a life centered on food to come out. They do not have to make excuses for being large or obsessed with food, they have a chance to be honest about the painful calculations they make every time food passes through their mouths, and the terror they face every morning wondering whether it is going to be a "good day" or a "bad day." They do not have to pretend they eat like a bird. They get a chance, possibly, for the first time ever, to discuss their eating openly and to explore the complicated feelings they may have about their bodies. For everyone in the group, it is possibly the first place they have been in which they feel they do not have to apologize for existing in the first place. Above all, the group offers help in getting through a problem that may seem insoluble on your own.

Beyond breaking the isolation there are, in addition, several other ways in which the group method can be beneficial. Within the group everyone has the same problem and so, although the compulsive eating is the reason which draws everyone together, in that assembling, the group can provide a means for a shift in the self-definition for individual members. What I mean by this is that by being in a group that accepts the part of one that is a compulsive eater—one can move beyond this limited concept of the self as a compulsive eater. As one can begin to see other compulsive eaters or fat women as having other attributes apart from the fat and can begin to see that fat has nothing to do with other values such as beauty, creativity, energy or caring, one can begin to see these attributes in oneself.

For example, when group member Joy can see
another member, Mary, as a kind, quick and tough
woman then Joy can look beyond her own
self-definition as a fat person and see that she has
additional qualities too. She can then begin to
extend her view of fat so that it does not
automatically trigger a response of repulsion or
rejection. Fat can then be seen as one of a number of
adjectives that can be coupled up with other
adjectives—beautiful, gracious, horrid, awful, polite, nice or generous. The fat is seen as just a part of
oneself, not the singular most defining characteris-
tic. People are more than any of their parts or even
the sum of their parts. If you have a big stomach on
which you focus, you are nevertheless more than
just a big stomach. However, if you have been
defined by others or have defined yourself solely as
someone of a particular size—and this definition
has had negative connotations, as is the case with
the adjective "fat"—then it is hard for that part of
yourself not to seem overwhelming. Expanding
your definition of self to include other qualities in
addition to the fat is crucial. This is so because at the
point of giving up the fat you are then not throwing
out all of yourself (a common fear) because you are
more than the fat. Joan felt that her fat was the only
thing she had in life that was all hers. She held on to
her extra weight tenaciously, fearing that if she lost
it, if she were to give up her fat, there would be no
essential Joan left. The group was extremely
important to her because she was forced to look at
herself through others' eyes—others who accepted
her size and sought additional characteristics in
defining her. She recognized the uniqueness of
others in the group, the particular configuration of

their personalities which made them the people they were. She could see how they retained these characteristics at varying weights during the course of the group, and she was thus able to see her own essential uniqueness and individuality, not predicated on her fat.

In addition, the group serves other important functions. The fat conveys messages to the outside world. For example, many women say when discussing self-assertion that they do not know how to say "yes" or "no" directly. They have the fantasy that their fat is doing it for them. In the context of the group, where everyone's fat means something different, it is starkly demonstrated that having the fat speak for you does not necessarily get the message across. Of course, in the case of unassertive behavior outside the group, the fat rarely succeeds in the job it is meant to do either, but the fantasy can cling. Within the group, not only *can* one begin to express oneself more directly but one *has* to. Without specific articulation the magical meaning of the individual's fat will never come through. Group members can support each other in their attempts to make the exchange—you have a forum for trying to use your mouth to speak and say what you are wanting, feeling or thinking instead of continuing to hope that the fat is doing it for you. Taking risks of this nature is often easier in groups. Group members who experience themselves as particularly unassertive can use the group to try out ways of asserting themselves. Group members can provide accurate feedback and encouragement. In a one-to-one situation the feedback is, of necessity, more limited.

When talking about images of thinness, some

women have expressed the fantasy that "When I am thin I will be competent, attractive, together, in good relationships... perfect." Group members can help each other challenge such unreal expectations—they can demonstrate from their own past histories of times when they were thin that life was not wonderful and easy all the time. This can then aid others in giving up such notions of perfection which rely on a race against oneself in which one is bound to lose. But perhaps more instrumentally, it is likely that group members will be of varying sizes and that there will be one or two women who represent the ideal weight of others in the group. These women, the compulsive thins, so to speak, have kept the problem within physical bounds and are as thin as the culture demands its women to be. Despite this, they have not found that in thinness everything in their life runs smoothly, and this can be an enormously helpful lesson to those who imagine that being thin means that everything will be fine. Losing weight then can be seen as just that, rather than heralding a whole transformation of one's life.

As well as helping women redefine themselves, the group is also valuable in providing a direct way of dealing with compulsive eating itself. Within a compulsive-eating group the focus of attention is always on what is the fat or thin expressing in one's life at the moment, or in one's past or in the here and now of the group. It is as though the protective functions of the fat, by being discussed and explored in the group, lose their power within that group and members have to search for new ways to protect themselves without relying on the weight. This then provides a learning experience in which group

members can see that they have other protective
mechanisms apart from the fat. This makes giving
up the fat much less scary.

Inevitably, during the life of a group, people are
at different sizes at different times. It can thus be
noted that one can lose weight and nothing
necessarily terrible happens. For example—Jill and
Margot, who were different sizes, both feared their
own "promiscuity" if they were to lose weight. In
both their cases their thin periods were times of
intense sexual activity. In the course of the group
both realized how scary these thin/sexual experiences had been and knew that before losing weight
again they would have to promise themselves that
hectic sexual activity did not automatically accom-
pany being thin. Margot lost a good deal of weight
first. She continued to reassure herself that she
could be thin and not express her sexuality as long
as she was scared. Meanwhile, Jill began to
incorporate sexuality into her life, so that she gave
up the idea of leaving sex only for thin times and
then scaring herself with her sexual interest when
slim. As Jill noticed Margot's new-found sexual
selectivity she was very encouraged. She could see
that sex was no longer bound up with weight in a
deprivation/binge model of "too fat to fuck" or
"thin and promiscuous." For Jill and Margot then,
each other's actions spelled important lessons. Jill
saw that someone with whom she strongly identified
could achieve something that had previously
seemed so impossible—Margot had lost weight
without becoming promiscuous. Similarly, Margot
learned from Jill that it was possible to be sexual at
any weight. This was particularly comforting
because Margot wished to get pregnant and had

connected many of her fears of pregnancy and
motherhood with the idea that she would not be
able to have sex if pregnant because she would be so
large that she would be sexually undesirable. Jill's
ability to be sexually involved at a higher weight
than either had thought possible helped Margot
recast her ideas about sexuality and size. She could
see that Jill's size did not indeed preclude her from
being sexual and attractive and she was heartened
by this.

There are other important aids that emerge from
working in a group setting which will become
obvious as I detail a self-help model. At this point,
though, I should like to spell out a few suggestions
to help a group start.

It is my experience that the number of people in a
group should not be too small. An optimum group
would have between five and eight members. Since
it seems to take a while for a group to stabilize its
membership—a few people always tend to drop out
or move away—initially it is a good idea to form
with slightly more than the number you desire. Age,
size or cultural background seem to make little
difference to the outcome of the group. Of course
the similarity or difference in these factors will get
expressed in the flavor and feeling of any particular
group.

It is important to have a set length to the group
session, one that does not vary from week to week.
About 2½ hours makes sense for an eight-person
group, or 1½ hours for a five-person group. A
prescribed time is important for a couple of reasons.
First, as in any therapy group, it designates those
particular hours during which the group will
purposefully focus on the psychological issue at

hand. The session time should not be vague because the issue of definition—beginning and end—is a particularly critical one for compulsive eaters in all respects. Second, if the time is clearly defined then each member is likely to attempt to get her needs met from the group in a systematic way. This will cut into the feelings of insatiability and dissatisfaction that many compulsive eaters experience. These sessions then take on the additional significance, since an allotted time out of the daily routine of things is devoted to them. They become the time in the week that is guaranteed for reflection and exploration.

It is likely that everyone will come to the group with the expectation and desire that participation will produce dramatic and instant weight loss. While it is hard to banish such thoughts, it must be emphasized that weight loss is not the immediate goal. The aim of the group is to break the addictive relationship toward food, and the guidelines that follow point to that end. In achieving this goal the group will find it helpful to approach the problem on two levels simultaneously. One level is the exploration of the symbolic meanings of fatness and thinness for the individuals in the group. On the second level we work on new ways to approach food and hunger. But before moving into the specifics of the first few meetings, an important aside on what I understand about psychological processes.

Any symptom such as compulsive eating has occurred for a good reason. We do not produce symptoms unless we have no other routes to express distress. It is not wise to attempt to remove symptoms without providing insight into their origin and purposes. In addition, unless alternative strategies are developed for dealing with the conflicts that the symptoms were protecting an individual could feel quite helpless. This could lead to a hazardous situation in which, in an extreme case, the individual develops a new symptom. If we just remove a symptom, like compulsive eating, we are then not only devaluing it, in effect, saying it was just a bit of craziness that needed surgical removal, we are also risking—precisely because of its importance—a "symptom switch." It is not particularly helpful to give up compulsive eating one week to be hit by a new symptom (such as insomnia or anxiety) some time later. What I am suggesting here is that anxiety may occur if a woman begins to do all sorts of things she imagined she would do when thin without having sorted out what it is that worries her in those situations. Without the weight to rely on she may feel undefended and scared. If she is no longer eating to assuage these feelings and cannot contain them, she may well convert them into anxiety. I am using anxiety here to express a severe state of unease and helplessness, in which an individual is seemingly incapable of intervening on her own behalf.

Anxiety is a reaction to a feeling that is unacceptable, frightening or overwhelming. The individual finds the anxiety, however troublesome, safer than the tolerance of the trigger emotion or event. For example, Sara was extremely frightened by her angry feelings, imagining that they could kill her. She worried that if she allowed herself to come into contact with her anger for more than a split second, her rage would overpower her family and friends and wipe them out. This fantasy is quite common among women and is largely due to the taboo against the open expression of female fury. Sara then got frightened by her own anger and instead of being able to sit with the fantasy she became anxious. The diagram below may help to explain this process.

When Sara could accept that exploring her fantasy did not mean that she would carry it out—just because she felt like attacking all and sundry it did not mean she would—she no longer became anxious. She sat with her anger, it came and went and she felt in charge of it.

This digression about anxiety helps to explain how a rapid rejection of the compulsive eating can

UNACCEPTABLE ANGRY FEELING CREEPS INTO SARA	FANTASIES OF ACTIVE RAGE TO OTHERS	SARA GETS FRIGHTENED AT HER RAGE	SARA HAS A REACTION TO THE FRIGHT. NO LONGER FEELS THE ANGER	SARA IS ANXIOUS AND IS DISTANCED FROM HER TRUE FEELING

produce the same alienated symptom elsewhere unless sufficiently explored and incorporated. So I am concerned here to stress a few points:

1. Giving up the fat is a gradual process with emotional work being done at the same time.

2. The scary aspects of giving up the fat need to be faced.
3. Alternative ways of coping must be instituted.
4. Conflicts related to the eating and weight must be exposed.

These cautions are not, however, meant to suggest that it is necessary to restructure the whole personality before a symptom—such as compulsive eating—can be dissolved. It is our experience that, following the above lines, compulsive eating can be given up and that in learning to take care of oneself in the area of food an enormous self-confidence ensues.

When starting self-help groups we adopt the following structure for the initial meeting. The time is divided into two parts with the first half devoted to a preliminary exploration into the symbolic meanings of fat and thin for individual women. The second part is devoted to a discussion about food. Since you will presumably be doing this without a group leader it may be helpful for one group member to tape in advance the fantasy exercise that follows so that all members can participate during group time. If you do decide to tape it, leave good pauses where the dots are. The whole exercise should take around 15 minutes to read. Group members are asked to hold all the images in their heads during this time after which they will share their experiences with each other.

Get as comfortable as you can.... Close your eyes... and imagine yourself at a party.... You are getting fatter... you are now quite large.... What

*does it feel like?... Take a note of your surround-
ings.... How do you feel about them?... What kind
of party is it?... What kinds of activities are going
on?... Notice whether you are sitting or standing,
or moving about.... What are you wearing and how
do you feel about your clothes?... What are they
expressing?... Observe all the details in this
situation.... How are you interacting with the other
people at the party?... Are you on your own or
talking, dancing, eating with others?... Do you feel
like an active participant or do you feel
excluded?... Are you making the moves to have
contact with others or are the other people at the
party seeking you out?... Now see what this "fat"
you is saying to the people at the party.... Does it
have any specific messages?... Does it help you out
in any way to be fat in this situation?... See if you
can go beyond the feelings of revulsion you might
have to locate any benefits you see from being this
size at the party.... Now imagine all the fat peeling
and melting away and in the fantasy you are as thin
as you might ever like to be... you are at the same
party.... What are you wearing now?... What do
these clothes convey about you?... How do you feel
in your body?... How are you getting on with the
other people at the party?... Do you feel more or
less included now?... Are people approaching you
or are you making the first moves?... What is the
quality of your contact with others?... See if you
can locate anything scary about being thin at the
party... see if you can get beyond how great it feels
and notice any difficulties you might be having with
being this thin.... Now go back to being fat at the
party... now thin again.... Go back and forth*

between the two images and particularly notice the differences.... When you are ready, open your eyes....

Now go around the room and share your fantasy. You will find that describing it in the present tense helps make the experience more vivid. For example, "In my fantasy I'm at a beach party, it's a very hot day and I'm wearing a terry-toweling robe over my swimsuit, trying not to draw attention to myself, I feel very awkward...." Do not worry if people's fantasies are both widely divergent and contradictory; the similarity of themes will emerge in due course. Be sure to use "I," in order to give each person space to describe her experience in her own words. Generalizing from individual experience can cause unnecessary friction if done prematurely. The exercise introduces in a concrete way the concepts outlined in the book. Inevitably, you will discover huge differences in your self-image fat and thin. You may find, for instance, that in the fat fantasy you are sitting chatting with another person while in your thin fantasy you are a sparkling wit and very much the center of attention; or you may be on your own while fat and dancing with everybody when thin. In particular, the thin images may correspond to the popular conception of thinness discussed before, or your own experiences of being thin. In discussing your fantasies, bear in mind the kind of person you feel that you must/will become when thin. After you have sat with the image for a while see how it corresponds to your personality. Is the thin you a foreigner or, as some women comment, so decidedly different from your habitual self-image that you feel that you have two distinct personalities—fat and thin.

In our group, we raise the following questions both in the initial meeting and in subsequent meetings because it goes to the very heart of the issue of how to find other means of protecting yourself which work as well as weight:

1. What of myself that emerged in my fat fantasy must I promise to take with me thin?
2. What did I find scary in my fat fantasy so I can promise myself I do not have to do it when I get thin?

In the fantasy, one group member, Maureen, was sitting with another person when fat, and had become a sparkling wit thin. As she explored the qualities associated with these two different states she remarked on the safety and ease she felt chatting with her friend as compared to the driven and insecure quality associated with the sparkling wit. By recognizing the negatives associated with thinness and the benefits of fatness, Maureen saw that, in order for her to lose weight permanently, she must allow herself the possibility that a thin her would not necessarily want to sparkle incessantly. She saw that her view of thinness, while superficially pleasurable and rewarding, was at great variance with her concept of her fat self, and that losing weight did not mean a complete personality change. Neither was the latter possible or desirable. Sparkling all the time for someone who enjoys relaxed conversation is unrealistic. *It is precisely this changed concept of self that puts the weight back on because it is enormously stressful trying to be someone entirely different when thin.* So Maureen had to promise herself that if she were to lose the weight she would not also have to lose the part of her that enjoyed relaxed chatting. She had to consider the possibility that her desire to chat, for example, was not an attribute of her fat but an aspect of her personality. Similarly, she had to consider that the part of her that wanted to be a sparkling wit did not have to wait to emerge until she were thin. Being overweight does not preclude one from being "the star." It does not mean one always has to be backstage waiting for thinness to bring you forth.

I have used Maureen's example for two reasons; not only because of the frequency with which it comes up, but also to delineate the line of questioning to pursue. Obviously not everybody will find such a clear-cut discrepancy between a fat self-image and a thin self-image at an initial meeting. The fantasy exercise provides a way for the compulsive eater to enrich her view of what fat and thin mean to her. Then we can go on to ask what kinds of unreal expectations are attached to thinness, and what we imagine we shall be giving up in getting there. These questions are ones that need to be continually raised in the group and help to develop a self-image that does not vary with body size.

After everyone has shared their fantasies and, perhaps, seen common threads, we move on to consider the technical work of the group on ways to approach food and hunger. We do another fifteen-minute fantasy trip which aims to highlight current feelings toward food at the same time as suggesting new possibilities. Tape this or delegate one person to read it while the group gets as comfortable as possible:

Close your eyes.... Now I should like you to imagine you are in your kitchen.... Look around the room and make a note of all the food that is in it... in the refrigerator... closets... cookie tin... freezer.... It probably is not too hard for you to form a complete picture because undoubtedly you know where everything is or is not, including any goodies or dietetic foods.... Look around the room and see how it is affecting you.... Is it painful to see how pathetic the foods are that you generally keep there or allow yourself to eat?... See what your kitchen says about you.... Now go to your favorite supermarket or shopping mall or a place where there is a wide variety of stores under one roof—greengrocer, butcher, delicatessen, dairy, bakery, take-out food store—and I should like you to imagine that you have an unlimited amount of money to spend.... Take a couple of supermarket carts and fill them up with all your favorite foods.... Go up and down the aisles or from counter to counter and carefully select the most appetizing foods.... Be sure not to skimp... if you like cheesecake, take several, take enough so you feel that there is no way you could possibly eat it all in one sitting... be sure to get the specific ones you really like.... There is no hurry, you have plenty of time to get whatever you want.... Cast your eyes over the wonderful array of foods and fill up your cart.... Make sure you have everything you need and then get into a cab with your boxes of food and go to your home.... There is nobody in the house

*and nobody will be around for the rest of the day,
the house—especially the kitchen—is all yours for
you to enjoy. . . . Bring the food into the kitchen and
fill up the room with it. . . . How do you feel
surrounded by all of this food just for you? . . . Does
it feel sinful, or is it a very joyful feeling? . . . Do you
feel reassured or scared by the abundance of food
just for you? . . . Just stay with the food and go
through the various moods that come up . . .
remember nobody will disturb you, the food is there
just for you, enjoy it in whatever way you want
to. . . . See if you can relax in the knowledge that you
will never again be deprived. . . . And now I should
like you to go down the road to mail a
letter. . . . How do you feel about leaving the house
and all the food? . . . Does it give you a warm feeling
to know that when you go back it will still be there
for you undisturbed? Or is it a relief to get away
from it? . . . You have now mailed the letter and are
on your way back to the house. . . . Remember as
you open the door that the food is all there just for
you and no one will interrupt you. . . . How does it
feel to be back with the food? . . . If you found it
reassuring before does it continue to be so? If you
found it scary can you find anything comforting in
being in the kitchen with all this food? . . . Slowly
come back to this room here with the knowledge
that your kitchen is full of beautiful foods to eat that
nobody is going to take away from you . . . and,
when you are ready, open your eyes. . . .*

Responses to this fantasy trip vary enormously
but, as you will find, it rarely generates anything but
dramatic reactions. These range from huge feelings
of relief at having so much food available and the

permission to enjoy it, to horror, fright and worries about one's ability actually to be in a room with all that food, from urges to throw it away or throw it around the room, to even lying in it. For many women, the trip to the mailbox provides much-needed relief from the claustrophobic feeling of being surrounded by "tempting" foods; for others, it is a serene break from a kitchen that has been transformed into a beautiful nurturing environment. The fantasy pinpoints our deeply held worries about food and provides a good starting point for a discussion about just how much compulsive eaters deprive themselves of the enjoyment of food and just how much food has been converted into an enemy. In conveying a permissive idea toward food we are attempting to make inroads into the conception that because one is a compulsive eater or overweight, one must deprive oneself of food. The central idea to be conveyed is, in fact, precisely the opposite and it rests on a challenge to the premise that a compulsive eater never really allows herself to eat. She is always acting out of a model that says, "I'm too fat, I must deny myself certain foods." This sets up a paradigm in which she is either dieting or eating a lot of food in preparation for tomorrow's diet, when she must be "good." The diet is invariably broken by a binge hardly enjoyed because of its driven and stolen quality. Then follows a period of "chaotic eating" and eventually a new diet plan as the chart below illustrates. None of this kind of eating contains within it a positive attitude toward food but rests on a frenetic struggle to control one's food intake.

This continual struggle to control one's food intake is a propelling factor in compulsive eating.

The aim of our method is to redefine, for the compulsive eater, both the function of food and her entitlement to it. *People need food in order to live. Food is a life-giving source and not something to be avoided.* As long as there is plenty, food can be

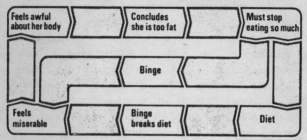

Feels awful about her body → Concludes she is too fat → Must stop eating so much

Binge

Feels miserable ← Binge breaks diet ← Diet

enjoyed. This idea, while hardly revolutionary, sounds staggering for someone who has been using food for other purposes. In due course I will discuss ways to implement this method but what is important in the first meeting is that group members share their daily experiences and fears about food.

This then, is the outline for the first meeting. Subsequent sessions will benefit from continuing work on the two levels—people's experiences with food that week and themes in relation to fat and thin although the time for doing this need not be structured so rigidly. The self-help groups that we have started take away a homework assignment for the first week—to keep a food chart. The purpose of this chart is to sort out some of the themes that continually reappear for you when you find yourself going toward food when you know you are not physically hungry.

Keep a record along these lines for the first week. The point of the chart is to *observe* how you eat and not to judge it. Through the entries on the chart you

can begin to get a sense of what kind of eating
patterns emerge for you. Do you experience
yourself eating chaotically or with some consistency? Did any foods taste particularly satisfying?
How does it feel to realize that your food intake is so
circumscribed by "shoulds?" Wasn't the chocolate
cake and ice cream at three o'clock in the morning
much tastier than the spinach and fish at regulation
suppertime? Come on, wasn't it really a drag to eat
that hamburger and salad in order to get to the
ice-cream sundae you really wanted?

TIME & DAY	WHAT I ATE	WAS I HUNGRY BEFORE EATING?	DID FOOD SATISFY ME OR NOT?	FEELINGS PRIOR TO EATING

In addition to discovering what the chart reveals
about actual food intake, it is also helpful to look at
the circumstances in which you habitually eat. Do
you eat alone? in hiding? never making dates to see
people around traditional mealtimes? or do you eat
with "eating friends" in restaurants? or at home at a
table? or at home walking around your house or
apartment, half in the refrigerator? or in bed? or
watching television? Observe when, how and what
you eat, and when, how and what you enjoy the
most. It may be that you will find that eating alone
so absorbs you that it is nicest to sit yourself down at
a beautifully set table, or you may find that you like

a multi-media show with book open, music playing
and the food in the middle.

Notice too the entries under "Feelings prior to
eating." Is there any consistency in what triggers the
eating when you are not particularly hungry? Can
you pinpoint specific emotions which you find hard
to cope with that drive you toward the refrigerator?
In our groups many women mention boredom,
anger, feelings of emptiness, disappointment, and
loneliness as triggers. For others, the eating is like a
punctuation point between various activities with
the food marking the beginning and end of different
phases of the day. Other women notice that they eat
to give themselves a treat. The food provides—
albeit fleetingly—an oasis of pleasure in an
otherwise difficult day. As Isabel put it, "If I didn't
know I was going to have a few cream donuts during
the day I couldn't see how I'd get access to pleasure."
In exploring this remark of hers, she dealt with
several issues. Why was her life structured in such a
way as to preclude other "accesses to pleasure?"
What does pleasure mean to her? Is she entitled to
it? If she waits for others to give to her is she risking
not getting? Must she therefore control it to ensure
that she gets it? What other things would she enjoy
as much? Does she always want cream donuts when
she is hungry for pleasure or are there other
pleasure-giving activities as well? These questions
are raised in the service of examination. Isabel is not
encouraged to give up her cream donuts. Quite the
contrary, the aim of the group is to help her to enjoy
her food more consistently so that every time she
eats she is having a treat—it is a waste of an eating
experience not to eat something really tasty. Isabel
is encouraged by the group to think about her

concept of pleasure and the immutability of her belief that no one but herself could possibly please her. This behavior, while essential to her, was also a protection against her fear that others would inevitably disappoint her—let her down. Providing her own treats made her less vulnerable while she imagined that her fat kept the world away. This difficulty over pleasure is a familiar one for many women and speaks poignantly to the pain with receiving that they experience.

It is on this level that questions need to be raised. In the first few sessions, as you are getting to know each other, gentle inquiries will help elicit useful information both about group members' behavior and the motivations behind it. Apart from discussing the food chart at the second meeting (and incidentally the chart can be used from time to time to help you check in with what you have been eating and how), you might start to go around the room and share your weight histories with each other. What is important here is not how many pounds you were at a particular point but the circumstances of your life through various weight changes. Notice any particular periods when your weight increased, using a family photo album to jog your memory if you find that helpful. Most likely, your group will include people with a range of stages in weight gain, including childhood, adolescence, leaving home, marriage, divorce, pregnancy or when the kids leave home. Leave yourself plenty of time to go through these histories, extending them over several sessions if necessary, so that you capture both the details and the quality of your own past relationship to your body and food. Make sure that you discuss your family's involvement with your food intake. Did/

does anybody else in the family have an eating problem? What were the unspoken rules and regulations about food? What was the significance of mealtimes in your family? Were meals a harmonious time or very strained? Was there enough food in the house or were certain foods banned and only eaten away from home? Did your mother help you to diet or did she discourage your attempts? Did your husband egg you on to reduce or "tempt" you with forbidden foods whenever you were actually dieting? Were there confusing messages from those close to you about how thin or fat you should be? Did you feel you had to be thin for someone else?

As the group continues and you become involved in trying to determine your own food intake, notice how the significant people in your life continue to play a role in relation to you and food. You may notice that your preoccupation with food has extended to hooking them into your eating behavior so that they either actually are judges or you imagine them to be so. It will be very important for you to be the only one in charge of your eating from now on. This will mean:

1. Disentangling yourself from when and what others wish to eat.
2. Daring to believe that you can begin to take care of your own eating.
3. Getting rid of the person to whom you designated the role of judge.

If your lover has been roped into helping you not to eat "bad foods" in the past and when you have sat down for supper together, his or her presence has stopped you gorging, reclaim that power for yourself but this time not in order to keep you away from the dangerous activity of eating but in the interest of helping you discriminate and select the foods you really enjoy.

Many people I have worked with have realized that their husbands have encouraged them to eat a lot while at the same time proclaiming their interest in slim, trim bodies. This was not dissimilar to their mothers' attitudes—an insistent "Eat, eat, child," or "A spoonful for Auntie Jane," or "Just one more bite for the poor starving kids in Europe!" These phrases were uttered with such pity and urgency that rejection was almost impossible even though the children were ready to gag. Rejection of the food felt like the rejection of mother. At other times, the same mothers beseeched their daughters to watch what they were eating lest their figures be ruined, or attempted to limit the food when they were larger than the "acceptable" size.

Pull out as much information as possible about past eating patterns and how they relate to your present experiences with food. For those women who were *schtupped* (over-fed) by their mothers, consider what goes through your mind when you feel too full to have another mouthful but still cram in extra food. What would it mean to you to stop at the point of fullness? As you meander back and forth between your own past and present experiences with food, bear in mind that we are trying to challenge the idea that the compulsive eater is not entitled to food. Our view is that compulsive eaters are terrified of food (once having invested it with magical properties—for instance, comfort against loneliness, boredom, anger or depression—it is hard to see it as just food, a source of nourishment) and are constantly eating or avoiding eating in response to this terror. Just because you feel out of control when near food does not mean you are not entitled to eat.

Many women say that being in charge of their own food strikes them as particularly difficult because although they have been responsible for feeding others they feel that in the one area in which they could take responsibility for themselves they have abdicated it. They are worried that they will not dare or even know how to be that self-concerned. It is important to remember that while compulsive eating feels like an abdication it is, nevertheless, a definite act for which one has been responsible. The meanings behind the compulsive eating may be unclear so that you are left with feelings of being out of control or at the mercy of the food, but this is the conscious experience and at the unconscious level the activity has a purpose. If you can think of converting that responsibility for your food into a concerted effort to notice when you are hungry and what kinds of foods you are wanting, you will be able to approach many social situations which involve food with more confidence. Some common fears that come up in the groups involve practical issues, for instance, how to ensure your own food supply when living with others. In the group, it will be useful to explore the actual situation. Is it a family group, a commune, or roommates? Is food bought and eaten together, is suppertime the only time the household congregates? From this kind of information, alternatives will come. These may include keeping a shelf in the

refrigerator of foods just for yourself and asking
other household members to replace immediately
any foods they take; withdrawing from the com-
munal shop or allowing yourself a certain amount
of money each week for food over the household
budget so that you ensure you are getting what *you*
want; explaining to household members that you
have had a painful time around food and are trying
to learn your body's real needs. Consequently, you
may eat in a rather unorthodox way and would they
please refrain from comments and cajoling. Another situation which frequently crops up is going to
someone's house for supper. Group members often
express alarm at this situation. We suggest several
possible strategies: not to make social engagements
at mealtimes for a while where you cannot choose
what food is available; if it is a close friend the odds
are that she or he has lived through several diets
with you and been subjected to your instructions
about permissible foods before. If this is the case
you will benefit by telling your friend that your new
interest in food may lead you to not eat everything
on your plate and you hope they will understand. If
you get hungry an hour or so before it is time to go,
eat just a little to respond to it. That way the hunger
will still be available to you an hour later. Above all,
remember that you are entitled to eat, however
awful you feel about yourself and your body. Just
because you have used food for other than
physiological reasons in the past, it does not mean
you are to deprive yourself from here on.

As the group progresses you will want to
incorporate the various exercises that are sewn
through the body of this book.

1. Mirror work—in which you are trying to build a center that includes the fat, pages 87–88.
2. Dressing for now—not waiting until you are thin to express yourself, pages 89–91.
3. Leaving food on your plate, pages 122–123.
4. Make your kitchen a supermarket, pages 145–146.

The above exercises will heighten your awareness of your body and help toward a self-acceptance. As I have stressed before, ownership of your whole body, including the fat, is a crucial factor in preparing you for a life at a lower weight. It will be very important for you to feel that your body has power at whatever size and that you can communicate through how you use it. An issue raised frequently throughout this book is how women imagine that their fat keeps people away. It is almost as though their fat is walking in front of them announcing their self-loathing to the world. We are aiming to build confidence to keep people away (if that is what is wanted) which rests on a self-acceptance rather than a self-disgust. The more you are your body, the more you can say "no" with the whole of you. The fat then loses one of its functions as the ability to fend people off gets attributed to *you* and not solely to the fat. To help increase your acceptance and knowledge of your body you might begin to think of it as not simply a stomach or a mouth but an organic whole.

Try to experience the continuity in your body; feel it as one whole. You might try drawing unsigned pictures of yourselves within the group which can then be passed around for people to guess who is who. Since most group members will tend to represent themselves inaccurately, particularly in the early stages of the group, other members can provide help in correcting these perceptions by giving feedback about the poses, proportions and stances illustrated in the drawings. Polaroid photos can also be used to provide insight into how one projects oneself. As you become more and more familiar with your body you will be able to throw out your scales. The scales are yet another of those external measures of how well you are doing. Compulsive eaters are frequently hooked on scales. Every morning or night there is the ritual of evaluation; one finds out whether one has been "good" or "bad." The pounds of wisdom have in the past given one the right either to binge or to starve. In general, for the compulsive eater, the scales are the real judge. If you have done well (lost weight) then the scales allow you to eat. If you have done badly (gained weight) the scales throw you into a depression only relieved by a binge or a plan to lose the weight yet again. So, instead of this twice-daily torture with its concomitant anxieties, we try to develop a familiarity with our bodies so that the feelings can come from the inside rather than the outside. The scales have become another outside evaluator which women can afford to do without.

The mirror exercise can help us move toward self-validation (a hard struggle indeed against the messages in women's magazines about how we should look, feel and weigh) and begin to rely on our own senses of self. For particular parts of your body that give you trouble try doing the fat/thin fantasy exercise focused on that specific area. For example, if you feel tremendous hatred toward your thighs, imagine yourself with fat thighs and then with ideal

thighs and examine the meanings of the two
different body states. One woman I worked with
who longed for thinner thighs discovered in her
fantasy that the fat around her thighs was like a
house around her vagina. The concave thighs she
yearned for actually made her feel vulnerable as
though there was no protection against her
sexuality. Through the fantasy work she was able to
accept the "hated thigh fat" and see it as one way she
had coped with her sexuality. As she lost weight she
began to find other ways to express her interest or
lack of interest in sexual contact. For other women,
full breasts or stomachs have symbolized one thing
in conscious life but quite other meanings have been
revealed by doing the fantasy exercises. The insights
gained have empowered the women to review the
limited ways in which they have communicated with
their bodies. In the groups, or alone in front of a
mirror, you can experiment with projecting different aspects of your personality through your stance.
Try a variety of sexual expressions—project yourself as forceful, timid, retiring or active.

In preparing yourself for being thin without the
thin meaning "I must be wonderful, competent,
beautiful, clever," spend a few minutes during every
day on mundane tasks, imagining yourself thin
while doing them. This could be the ride to work,
social contact at work or home, going shopping or
waking up feeling thin. Particularly watch for
anything difficult about being thin in those daily
routines. If you find things scary try and investigate
just exactly what it is that is frightening and then
discuss these experiences within the group. Then try
feeling thin without associated elations and fears.
Notice how you would walk, stand or sit when thin

and try to incorporate those different poses into your body as you are now. If it is too long a jump, imagine yourself ten pounds lighter rather than dramatically thinner. This image may be more accessible and you may find less discrepencies in feeling the ten-pound difference. As this emerges it will mean that you are ready to lose some weight. Most likely, your body will indicate this by requiring less food. At these points, in particular, you will want to tighten up the process—being sure to eat exactly what you want and stopping precisely when you are full. Many compulsive eaters are unfamiliar with a full feeling that is not a bursting feeling. As an introduction to that bodily experience, eat several mouthfuls of whatever food you are wanting when you are hungry, being sure to taste them as they go down. Now leave the food for fifteen minutes and involve yourself with some other activity. After a quarter of an hour see how your body feels. If it feels hungry and empty, continue to eat whatever food you think will fit that hunger. If it feels comfortable it means you are quite full and you can wait until the next hunger signals to eat again. If you are sure that you will allow yourself to eat whenever you feel hungry, and that you will give yourself whatever kind of food it is that you are wanting, you will find that it is less necessary to stuff yourself. When your body then indicates that it is not wanting much food, it means it is time for you to lose a little weight.

People vary enormously but it has been my observation that in the early stages of the group, members tend to stabilize or gain slightly. For those who do gain weight, this should not be a signal for alarm but an opportunity to experience what the fat

is all about. It is a chance to embrace all the fat
before a final goodbye. As you lose weight you will
notice you may be inclined to lose a bit and then sit
there for a while. It is as though your body is holding
still while you do the next level of emotional work
exploring fantasies such as "Who will I be?" "Who
won't like it if I'm slimmer?" "How will I protect
myself if I am ten pounds lighter?"

In the previous chapters I have suggested that fat
has a lot to do with conflict about self-definition and
assertion and that a worry associated with being
thin is that one will be meek and mild and could be
blown over. Body work as described above will, of
course, help one live within one's body and thus use
it more instrumentally in day-to-day living but
additional homework exercises which strike at a
woman's often-felt unentitlement will also prove
helpful. These exercises are loosely grouped under
an assertion heading and flow from attempts to
define one's food intake.

Attempt to say "yes" to something you want
every single day. This could be something that only
involves you, for example, taking a bubble bath,
reading a book, going for a walk or writing a letter.
As you learn to say "yes" you will be fulfilling many
things. Primary among these is saying that you are
entitled to decide things for yourself. This in turn
produces a certain amount of self-confidence and
provides a chink in a self-image full of denial. As
you are able to say "yes" to a bath, so you will be
able to say "yes" to a snack when you want it. As you
learn to say "yes" you have the possibility of saying
"no." Think of an incident in which you said "yes"
but really wanted to say "no." Replay that incident
slowly in your mind's eye, only substituting "no"

and expressing the real feeling. Notice how that feels. What are you risking by saying "no?" Now be conscious of the many times you are in this situation. Begin to say "no" to things—even on what may seem like a minuscule level—as you begin to say "yes" to others. Develop the sense of feeling more in charge. This will flow over to the food—being able to say "yes" and to say "no" and, perhaps more centrally, will provide you with a new way to use your mouth in expressing yourself.

The fat/thin fantasy on pages 140–142 can be useful for discovering what different body sizes mean to individual group members in different circumstances. Topics you might find helpful to discuss are: What being fat and thin express for you living in this culture; what fat and thin have to do with sexuality, with anger, with competition, with your mother, with your father, or with your children. Add a specific person or situation to the one in the standard fantasy and draw out the issues as they occur for each person. For example, *"Get as comfortable as you can... imagine you are with your mother/father/husband...you are quite fat...."*

Now it may happen that in some groups only certain people talk or you may discover that the "fat" is working in the group in some of the same ways in which it operates outside the group. If a particular member has experienced a week of bingeing, then she might feel she has more of a right to group time: "If I am fatter, then I'm worse off than everyone else and I've a right to a lot of attention," or if a group member was consistently losing weight she might feel she does not have the right to group time: "If I am thin, then I'm supposed to be perfect and not have any needs." The woman losing weight might start to overeat in order to ensure her place in the group. If this situation crops up where those who have most difficulty that week get most time and those who have a relatively easy time with food are quiet, you might consider instituting a "twelve-minute rule," which means that each member is assured of twelve minutes of work time to discuss whatever she wishes in relation to food, fat or thin. This way you will be reinforcing neither fantasy—that thin, one has no needs and fat, one is insatiable.

In a self-help group, some people will play a more active role than others. However, it is the group as a whole that has responsibility for working together, selecting exercises, meeting places and times. You may find it helpful to rotate on a weekly basis so that a different person is in charge each time, preparing the exercises, keeping time and starting off the meetings. This is not essential, however, and every group develops its own patterns.

Self-help is an exciting concept in action. The potential to learn what is truly useful to you is enormous and, unhampered by preconceptions of what must or should happen, it opens the way for creative experimentation, evaluation and growth.

The guidelines above are to help you get going on the lines that our experience has shown to be useful, but they are in no sense intended to stifle the energy and imagination that you or your group feels to explore aspects of compulsive eating and self-image that are not addressed in detail here.

Self-starvation—
Anorexia nervosa

There is an elaborate and complicated eating condition closely related to compulsive eating called anorexia nervosa. It too, is characterized by self-imposed restrictions on food intake, a fear and terror of food and an obsessive—although secretive—interest in food. Unlike compulsive eaters, however, those who suffer from anorexia nervosa express their preoccupation with food by becoming very thin indeed—to the point of emaciation and sometimes even to the point of death through starvation. This extreme form of self-starvation is distinguished by a struggle to transcend hunger signals.

It often takes off from an exaggerated applica-
tion of a diet, started because the potential anorectic
feels fat. Like the compulsive eater, many anorectics
engage in large-scale eating binges. The shame and
self-disgust that follow propel an anorectic to fast,
vomit or take laxatives—to purge her body of the
food that has been taken in. When food is eaten
again, feelings of bloatedness occur very quickly so
food intake continues to be very minimal until
another explosion of seemingly uncontrolled gorging occurs. Weight loss can be very dramatic and, in
turn, creates a wide range of physical symptoms.
Anorectics do not menstruate, often suffer from
insomnia and constipation, hypersensitivity to hot
and cold, excess hair growth on the body, changes in
the color and texture of existing hair, nails and skin,
slow pulse rate and perspiration. These physical
discomforts are endured in an attempt to reach the
overriding aim—to become thin.

While the idea of an interest in becoming fat is
difficult to grasp, few people would have difficulty
in understanding this interest in becoming thin
because it conforms to social expectations for
women. It is also quite easy to understand that 90
percent of clinically diagnosed anorectics are
women and that one of the workers in the field[1]
argues that the definition of anorexia nervosa
should be reserved for a special clinical syndrome
occurring in pre-pubescent and pubescent girls.

It is the fact that anorexia nervosa is almost
exclusively a woman's condition that ties it so
closely to compulsive eating and obesity. For if men
were to suffer from the same problem to a similar
degree we should seek a different explanation. But
the fear of obesity, the obsession with food, the

hidden and furtive eating and the interest in feeding others, leads us to identify the behavior as having origins in the social conditions of women in our society. *Anorexia nervosa is the other side of the coin of compulsive eating. In her rigorous avoidance of food, the anorectic is responding to the same oppressive conditions as compulsive eaters.*

It is important to note that while I have had little direct experience with anorectics, many women who suffer with this problem have sought me out because in reading of the Munter-Orbach view of compulsive eating they have found much with which to identify. Thus, what I have to say will be based on my reading of the works[2] on anorexia nervosa and discussions with women who have had anorexia, rather than on long-term clinical experience. My interest in touching on anorexia in this book is insofar as it sheds light on compulsive eating which is at the other end of the continuum. A feminist interpretation of anorexia confirms the approach used in compulsive eating.

Both anorectics and compulsive eaters binge and starve themselves. However, the anorectic starves for long periods subsisting on as little as an egg and a cookie a day and only occasionally bursting out into a binge which is then purified by even more rigorous fasting or cleansing by laxatives, vomiting or enemas. This bird-like eating is a reflection of a culture that praises thinness and fragility in women. Many women pinpoint the onset of their anorexia as an exaggerated response to dieting and teenage ideals of femininity. As with compulsive eaters, sensing something amiss at adolescence, they sought the answer in their individual biology. Their bodies were changing, becoming curvy and fuller, taking on the shape of a woman. They were changing in a way over which they had no control—they did not know whether they would be small breasted and large hipped or whether their bodies would eventually end up as the teenagers in *Seventeen*.

These upheavals rendered in these young women feelings of confusion, fear and powerlessness. Their changing bodies were associated with a changing position in their worlds at home, at school and with their friends. A curvy body meant the adoption of a teenage girl's sexual identity. This is the time for intense interest in appearance, the time when girls learn the tortuous lesson about not revealing their true selves to boys whether on the tennis court or in school, or in discussing affairs of the heart. These new rules and regulations governing behavior, and the explosive changes taking place are quite out of tune with what has previously been learned and the feelings they generate are enormously complicated. Several women have said on looking back on this time in their lives—a time when they were growing and yet effectively stopped eating— that they felt so out of phase with all that was going on that withdrawal from food was an immensely satisfying way to be in control of the situation. In transcending hunger pangs they were winning in one area of the struggle with their apparently independently developing bodies. They were attempting to gain control over their shapes and their physical needs. They felt their power in their ability to ignore their hunger.

But this power to overcome hunger results in a contradiction because in her very attempt to be strong, the anorectic becomes so weak that she becomes less independent, more dependent. She needs more care and concern from others because of her weakened physical state. This adaptation poses yet another dilemma. As Rosie Parker and Sarah Mauger write, "For a great many women manipulation of their own bodies is too often their only means of gaining a sense of accomplishment. The link between social status and slimness is both real and imagined. It is real because fat people are discriminated against; it is imaginary because the thin, delicate ideal image of femininity only increases a person's sense of ineffectualness." [3]

This latter point is, perhaps, the crux of the matter. Anorexia reflects an ambivalence about femininity, a rebellion against feminization that in its particular form expresses both a rejection and an exaggeration of the image. The refusal of food which makes her extremely thin straightens out the girl's curves in a denial of her essential femaleness. At the same time, this thinness parodies feminine petiteness. It is as though the anorectic has a foot in both camps—the pre-adolescent boy-girl and the young attractive woman. This has its echoes too in compulsive eating. For some women who eat compulsively the excess weight is also an attempt to defeat the curviness of the female body which brings in its wake dreaded social consequences. Mary, who had a compulsive-eating problem, started to overeat when she became a teenager and explained with hindsight that she was trying to smooth out her curves. The "puppy fat" she acquired put her less in the girls' camp with the concomitant dating and beautifying rituals. She was able to see herself as one of the kids—rather than one of the potential dating partners. Pre-adolescence suggested a kind of equality to her, where kids were just kids and could do more or less the same things. Her fat was an unconscious attempt to hide her curves just as the starving anorectic attempts to disguise her form by ridding it of substance. In the ultra-feminine image of the petite woman that anorectics frequently project there is yet another parallel in the compulsive eater.

Some women's largeness conforms to another stereotype of woman, in this case the all-giving, nurturing, reliable, loving, caring, earth mother who excels in feminine skills of caretaking, food preparation and sensual hugs. This aspect of fat is for some women a relatively positive image to hold on to because it is at least an accepted image and smacks less of freakiness, but it is an image that in itself is problematic because it is the extension of the woman's reproductive capacity into the role of being mother to the world. Mothers of the world are forever feeding others and consequently get exceedingly hungry. Petite young ladies are admired and showered on—so goes the myth—and they do not need to take as much in, perhaps because they do not have to give so much out. Their success in womanhood lies in their being cared for and pampered by others and not in caring for and pampering others.

This attempt to balance both fronts, the ultra-femininity and rejection of femininity, is related to another aspect of the syndrome that has been given wide attention. This is the anorectic's intense energy and activity. This activity expresses itself in a compulsion to do well in school, excel at sports, and keep on the go at all costs. Many people will be familiar with the feeling of a second wind in the midst of an exhausting late night and the kind of tense energy this unleashes. It is a similar feeling to the hyperactivity that anorectics frequently feel for months and months on end. This rushing about is partly motivated by an overpowering desire to lose yet more weight by burning up as many calories as possible. A feminist viewpoint suggests an additional root cause. The young woman's attempt to be involved in as many activities as possible is a protection against the exclusion she anticipates on entering womanhood because, in projecting into her future, she sees that the world is made up of men who are rewarded for being out in the world and women who are either excluded from activity in the world or, even more devious, included but not rewarded. In her frantic activities and involvements it would appear that she is trying to give herself a broader definition than her social role allows. She is striving to make an impact in a world hostile to her sex. This intense activity is painfully mirrored in the response of some anorectics whose fragile sense of self leads them to withdraw from the public world into their rooms, thereby highlighting women's invisibility. For the compulsive eater the reflection is reversed. The outwardly super-efficient, confident fixer and doer who can handle anything and carries the world on her shoulders is the exaggeration of woman as breast to the world. At the same time it underscores a woman's invisibility. The immovable blob—a common fantasy that compulsive eaters talk of—is analogous to the anorectic's intense activity and her experience of her self as ineffectual.

These converging images speak forcefully to a reconsideration of the origins of anorexia and as we

have already seen, compulsive eating. Previous
writers have emphasized some of the social factors.
Mara Selvini Palazzoli[4] suggests that the change
from an agrarian to an industrial society in Europe
has had a profound effect on the stability of the
patriarchal family and that the anorectic young
woman is a challenge to its continuing conserva-
tism. Hilde Bruch[5] addresses current social attitudes
toward body size and considers the extent to which
"the concept of beauty in our society, and our
preoccupation with appearance enter into the
picture. The obsession of the Western world with
slimness, the condemnation of any degree of
overweight as undesirable and ugly, may well be
considered a distorting of the body concept, but it
dominates present day living." Other social factors
such as Peter Dally's[6] observation that the mothers
of many anorectics were frustrated and hence
ambitious for their daughters are described but their
connection to the social situation of women in
society is not explored.

The pinpointing of these factors is extremely
helpful. However, there are still questions to be
answered. That is, why does this happen? Why is it
that some mothers are domineering? Why is
Western society preoccupied with slimness? Why
does the patriarchal family attempt to resist change?
What are the basic assumptions about our society
that women with eating disorders are challenging?
What in their abuse of the hunger mechanism and
their body distortions are these women gagging to
articulate how they feel? If this is a psychological
state that affects women, what is an appropriate
social response? Must not treatment include a
recognition of the social factors that lead women to

compulsive eating and anorexia nervosa?

As we have seen, modern Western societies place definite expectations and prohibitions on women's activities. Women are expected to be petite, demure, giving, passive, receptive in the home and, above all, attractive. Women are discouraged from being active, assertive, competitive, large and, above all, unattractive. To be unattractive is not to be a woman. In the case of compulsive eating, some women's strategy for dealing with these straitjacketed stereotypes is to become large to have bulk in the world; to become large to compensate for always giving out; to become large to avoid packaged sexuality. For the compulsive eater, food carries enormous symbolic meanings that reflect the problems women face in dealing with an oppressive social role. Even though anorectics have adopted the opposite strategy, self-starvation, the similarities to compulsive eating do not leave much doubt that the social position of women is as much reflected in the anorectic's behavior as it is in that of the compulsive eater.

Anorectics share with compulsive eaters a conscious desire not to be noticed. They often feel nervous walking into a room at a party lest all the attention is focused on them. Instead of gaining weight to hide a real self underneath the layers, the anorectic literally becomes paper thin. But this paper thinness attracts more attention than does a "normal"-sized woman. The crucial difference is that for emaciated (and overweight) women the interest they do attract is of a different nature than that which meets the woman of more "normal" size. The quick "once over" evaluation done by both men and women establishes the anorectic (and the obese

woman) as outside the status of a sex object.
Broadly, this means that men will dismiss her and
other women will relax in her presence. The
anorectic will be viewed as pathetic or regarded with
sympathy, but in her seemingly narcissistic striving
for ultra-femininity she curiously succeeds in
desexualizing herself. In addition, two related ways
to understand this worry about being noticed
suggest themselves. The first is reflected in the
repeated theme of women's invisibility—wafer
thinness is perhaps the quintessential expression of
women's absence/presence. This forced invisibility
leads in turn to a desire to be accepted and noticed
for just being, rather than for having to look and be
perfect and fulfill others' expectations. This desire,
strongly felt and rarely satisfied, has little option but
to be repressed, to be converted into its very
opposite—a fear of being noticed which in its
particular form makes the anorectic stand out.

This wish for acceptance stems, for many
women, from a feeling of unwantedness and hence
unworthiness. This may be either explicit: "We
really wanted a boy," or from a sensed disappointment the mother has in bringing a daughter into the
world. Whether explicit or implicit, the fact is that
many compulsive eaters and anorectics report
feeling their mothers expressed enormous ambivalence about their very existence. To say we were
hoping for a boy is to say to a daughter that she has
let you down. It is a short step from feeling that one
has fallen short of one's family's hope to feeling like
a failure. In its turn, failure can bring feelings of
non-entitlement. At puberty where it becomes
obvious that a girl is a girl, the feelings between
mother and daughter may become so acute that two

actions collide for the girl. She refuses food in an attempt to wither away, to not exist, to please her mother by disappearing. At the same time, the rage the daughter feels at not having been wanted for who she is, for not having had a mother with whom to identify—how can one identify with a mother who is self-rejecting without also adopting a rejecting self-image?—is expressed by a refusal to take in the one thing the mother consistently gives—food. In a mixture of rage and demureness, the adolescent girl gags on the first mouthful or is full after a few bites. She is rejecting what her mother gives and hurting her in the most powerful way she knows how while simultaneously carrying out what she imagines to be her mother's wish, which is for her to disappear.

The pressure that leads many parents to desire male babies is itself a consequence of living in a world that accords less social power to women. A tragic repercussion of women's inferior social position is that in the transmitting of culture from one generation to the next, the mother has the dreadful job of preparing her own daughter to accept a life built on second-class citizenship. It is in the learning of our gender identity—that is, what it means to be a girl and then a woman in this world—that we find our place in society. What defines this gender identity will vary widely in relation to class and cultural proscriptions so that what it means to be a woman factory worker in Bulgaria will be quite different than what it means to be a nurse in the United States but both these women will have become adults through conception of self, based on available models of feminine behavior, assimilated first from their mothers. It is

in the teaching of this gender identity that the
tensions in the mother-daughter relationship ex-
plode and the confusing messages of female
adulthood are incorporated by the young girl.

One aspect of this tension that seems especially
pertinent to anorectics is the concern with having
disappointed one's mother for having been a girl in
the first place. The girl feels she is a shaky second
best with a precarious right to survive. This worry
about the right to exist is also linked to the academic
excellence and performance aspects of anorexia.
Many women have reported that their need to excel
academically was a response to feeling that if they
should fail they would disappoint their parents. If
they did not disappoint their parents they might be
accepted—as one woman who suffered from
anorexia put it bitterly, "I had to perform. I wasn't
just accepted for who I was whereas my brother who
was a delinquent was!" In this woman's life there
was nothing explicitly stated about her not being
desired or wanted, it was rather a feeling she picked
up in relation to how she felt her brother was
treated. That they were treated differently just
because of their ages did not explain to her the
feelings she had about herself and her mother's
attitudes toward her. The only way she could
understand this vast difference in treatment and her
terribly painful feelings of being unaccepted was to
see it as part of her parents' disappointment with her
sex.

In the last thirty years, one of the most striking
differences between the upbringing of girls and boys
surfaced around adolescence when girls were
supposed to be pure and boys were supposed to
acquire sexual experience. Sex was definitely bad

for girls and good for boys. To girls it seemed as though boys could only win at this game: they either succeeded and became experienced or were reassured that there was plenty of time. Indeed, there was even a special category of women who provided boys with this experience. For the girls there was no way to win. If you did "it" you were bad, dirty, impure. Thinking about "it" was not much better either. If you did not do "it" boys would call you names, but if you did, you would get a bad reputation. You were preparing yourself for marriage many years hence and sexual activity up to that time was to be kept within definite limits. Against this background it is hardly surprising that young women are terribly confused about their sexuality, seeing it as evil, dangerous and explosive on the one hand and powerful, glorious and desirable on the other. Their sexuality becomes curiously disembodied from the person. It is an aspect of a young woman that in any event she must watch out for, almost as though it is some independent entity she must keep under control. This alienating view of sexuality from which women are now struggling to break free sheds much light on both the anorectic's and the compulsive eater's ambivalence about sexuality. The distortion of one basic body function gets carried over to another basic one, hunger. In the distortion of body size that follows, the manipulation of hunger feelings, the anorectic and the compulsive eater powerfully indict sexist culture. The young woman takes herself out of the only available sexual arena and worries that should she express her sexual feelings her whole world will crack.

In the retreat from a sexual identity the anorectic

young woman is pointing to the difficulties of the
various aspects of womanhood. Sexual identity is
an aspect of gender identity so that in rejecting
models of sexuality one is simultaneously rejecting
models of femininity. This is the dilemma that faces
many women and is expressed both through the
symbolic meanings of being thin and food refusal
for the anorectic.

For the anorectic then, the refusal of food is a
way to say "no," a way to reject. It is her way to show
strength. Her thinness, on the other hand, also
expresses her fragility and frailty, her confusion
about sexuality and her interest in disappearing.
For the compulsive eater the picture would seem to
be reversed with the fat expressing rejection,
protection and strength and the incessant consumption of food symbolizing capitulation. In both these
responses we see the adaptations to a female role
which has quite limited parameters. Both syn-
dromes express the tension about acceptance and
rejection of the constraints of femininity.

What is interesting in comparing these two
responses is to notice just where they converge and
where they differ. One area of striking difference
rests on the attitudes of those who suffer at either
end of the continuum. For the anorectic, her
problem is not a matter for public discussion. It is a
very private issue which she does not acknowledge
as a problem because she herself sees her refusal to
eat as an attempt to control her situation, a control
that feels precarious and that might be at risk if she
were to discuss it. This is quite different from the
experience of compulsive eaters who do not regard
their overeating as an active state but rather
something that happens only when they are out of

control. They are quite happy to discuss this exterior, invading force and often initiate conversation about their "problem." This can partly be explained by the fact that the social pressure to be thin is so great that compulsive eaters feel they must offer an excuse for their size. The anorectic, however fat she sees herself, is, in fact, conforming to society's demand for women to be thin.

Paradoxically, the general public takes anorexia nervosa quite seriously while viewing compulsive eating as the behavior of an overindulgent, greedy person. As we have seen, however, both activities are extremely painful responses to which women may turn in their attempts to have some impact in their worlds.

Medical issues

It is the thesis of this book that compulsive eating in women is a response to their social position. As such, it will continue to be an issue in women's lives as long as social conditions exist which create and encourage inequality of the sexes. Any treatment for overweight women must address this fact.

When a woman goes to see a general practitioner with a weight problem, the doctor will almost invariably tell her to go on a diet. In the doctor's eyes, it is clear that this patient eats too much and to lose weight she must eat less. This attitude is exactly the same as that implicit in all the diets thrown onto the market every day. The doctor has neither the time nor the interest to examine why this woman got fat in the first place. No dietary advice can help a woman lose weight permanently for the real reasons are not recognized and tackled.

Medical training today is becoming increasingly technical—high grades in scientific subjects have become essential to qualify for medical school and once there, the emphasis is on the technical approach to medicine. The human element of medicine is often lacking. This means that doctors are trained to make use of complex instruments and keep abreast of basic research. They do not acquire the sensitivity to recognize what is often troubling their patients. Therefore, many women are met with an unsympathetic face when they visit the doctor to lose weight. Doctors are no less susceptible than other people to cultural ideas about beauty and thinness and frequently feel entitled to comment on the size of their patient's body even when their medical problems are not related to it. As one woman put it, "They always make me feel guilty, like a naughty girl for eating too much." Clutching new diet sheets they are sent straight back to their homes and jobs and the problems they face there—the problems that were the main causes of their fatness in the first place.

But women come to know that diets and guilt do not work, whether they come from doctors or magazines. Some women may become desperate to find a physiological reason for their persisting fat. They may go further, to a specialist who deals with obesity and in whose interest it is to propose that there are biological factors which cause it. When a woman goes to a specialist she is seeking some further understanding; she may think "If there is a medical reason for my fat, then there is little I can do. I shall be fat but people should recognize that it is not my fault."

In recent years there has been considerable medical research into the causes of obesity. While few of these theories have been wholly absorbed into the practice of the medical establishment, the publicity they have received and the hope that they instill in overweight people leads me to discuss the most favored ones here.

Doctors and researchers with a mechanistic view of the human body picture it as an assembly of organs (liver, heart, brain), tissue (muscle, nervous tissue, bone), and cells (nerve cells, muscle cells and blood cells). Organs are composed of various kinds of cells, and the cells themselves are pictured as little biochemical factories that work to maintain the organism in good health. This perspective has allowed the development of a picture of obesity as a biological phenomenon. In the body there is tissue between organs like various muscle groups or bone and muscle, which is called connective tissue. This connective tissue has the capacity to accumulate fat that the body does not use. It is called adipose tissue and consists of cells which are called fat cells. It is in the pattern of accumulation of fat in the fat cells that has drawn the attention of many medical investigators.

THE FAT CELL THEORY Ten years ago Hirsch and Knittle[1] developed a method of counting the number and size of fat cells in a sample of adipose tissue. They suggested that obesity in childhood was accompanied by an increase in the number of fat cells in the body which are not reduced by dieting later in life. The cells themselves will reduce in size when a person loses weight but it is as though they are sitting waiting to be refilled. An extremely obese person can have as many as five times the normal number of fat cells. This theory is offered as an explanation for why some overweight people have difficulty keeping their weight down after dieting.

BIOCHEMICAL THEORIES The functioning of cells depends on the nature of chemical reactions which occur in them. All chemical reactions in the body—the conversion of food into energy, the expenditure of energy in exercise, indeed all human activity—depend on the presence of enzymes. Enzymes are protein molecules which assist the chemical reaction without being used up. Every chemical reaction in the body has an enzyme associated with it. Studies on bacteria have shown that the enzymes are made with the help of information stored in the genes. It is natural, therefore, from this perspective, to see a genetic explanation for obesity. Obese individuals are pictured as having slightly different genes from non-obese people. The different genes then result in slightly different enzymes. These enzymes are the ones that are involved in the chemical reactions related to the storage of fat in the body. The obese person is pictured as having different enzymes and hence their bodies respond to fat in a different way from the bodies of non-obese people.

GENETIC THEORIES Related to biochemical approaches is the genetic approach. The general genetic approach does not specify necessarily where the genetic variation occurs but simply hypothesizes that it exists, whether in the enzymes, the nervous system, or the hormonal system of the body. This approach leads to studies showing that "obesity runs in families."[2]

A new genetic theory[3] suggests that fat people do not necessarily eat more than thin people. The argument runs that in subsistence agricultural societies, the pattern of eating is feast and fast and that those with the ability to store excess energy efficiently and release it for physical labor have a better chance of survival. In affluent societies where there is a regular and adequate food supply there is not the same need for the body to store and release energy. Furthermore, since we tend to be more sedentary we burn off less excess energy. Computer simulation runs of the pattern of lean and fat deposition in adults are offered as evidence for a biologically determinist view that whereas until recently it was functional to have an inherent tendency toward fatness, nowadays it is functional to have a predisposition to thinness.

INSULIN-RELATED THEORY When sugar and protein are eaten the islets of Langerhans, which are cell clusters in the pancreas, produce the hormone insulin. Insulin is a vital protein that is necessary for cells to take in and utilize sugar as an energy source. If there is an excess of glucose in the bloodstream it is converted into stored energy or fat. If a body does not produce enough insulin, the sugar and carbohydrates accumulate in the blood and do not provide energy to maintain bodily processes and growth. This is diabetes. Two thirds of diabetics are obese and this has led researchers to question whether there is a link between the two conditions. The theory of hyperinsulinism conjectures that the body produces too much insulin which may itself induce insensitivity to the hormone.[4] It is this latter view that has been popularized by Dr. Atkins.[5] He calls insulin "the fattening hormone" and suggests that excess presence stimulates a person to eat more to maintain the balance. He sees insulin as the crucial link between overweight, low blood sugar and diabetes.

NEURAL THEORY Simple neural theory looks at the body's system of regulation. A region of the brain, the hypothalamus, has been conjectured to be the location where the body's messages about hunger are processed. A satiation center in the hypothalamus provides information on fullness. If there are lesions in this neural area, it is hypothesized, eating will continue beyond normal stopping point. A recent study on rats with ventromedial hypothalamus lesions which raise the set point, delay the onset of satiation and cause obesity, reported various motivational deficits including rats' failure to hoard. This failure to hoard has led the researchers to see a parallel in human motivation and they suggest that obesity causes poverty.[6]

Other researchers see the hypothalamus as less central to the regulation of hunger. The basic principle, however, remains the same. A defect in the body's regulation of hunger is hypothesized as being the cause of overeating.

The shortcoming of some of these theories is that they do not offer a way to determine whether observed differences in human reactions between obese and non-obese persons cause the obesity or are due to the obesity. The fat-cell theory has a limited use since a high proportion of fat cells in infancy occurs only with massive obesity. Treatment of adults who were obese as children does not prevent weight loss and stabilization.[7] General genetic theories suffer because observed family similarity fits equally with an environmental model.[8] The evolutionary functional theory is weakened by the authors' underestimation of the allowable rates of genetic change in time.[9] The hypothalamus lesion theory first describes rat behavior in human terms and in doing so falls into the trap of assuming that the observations of animal behavior are analogous to those of human behavior.[10]

What is most critical, however, are the treatment procedures which follow from these hypotheses. They offer the promise, through the understanding of human physiology of the development of a substance (a drug, for example), which can melt away excess fat cells, restore the satiation mechanism in the hypothalamus or permit the person's body to utilize more efficiently its fat and sugar intake. This attitude is to be seen in the treatment of diabetes. The body's inability to produce enough insulin is corrected by daily insulin injections. A similar treatment for compulsive eating or its usual effect—obesity—satisfies an often-expressed wish that the fat can be whisked away by a pill and we will be as thin as we like. The history of conflicting medical research into obesity for the last seventy-five years makes it unlikely that such a substance exists. Treatment that is often sought and used has commonly been focused on three major areas: drug therapy, surgical procedures, and diet therapy.

DRUG THERAPY One approach to deal with obesity has been to prescribe thyroxine, a hormone that is secreted by the thyroid gland. Thyroxine is supposed to "speed up metabolism" and in so doing causes the body to burn up food more rapidly. The long-term effects of this treatment are doubtful for it relies on very high dosages of the hormone. As such, it is potentially dangerous in that it can interfere with the body's normal thyroid functioning which is very delicate. Two other drugs are employed in the treatment of obesity. They are called anorectic agents. One class are appetite suppressants and known popularly as amphetamines or speed. The addictive and stimulative aspect of this drug has been well documented as has the patient's need for increased dosages to maintain a suppressed appetite. The other class are drugs such as Flenfluramine which aim to produce feelings of fullness and inhibit the synthesis of triglycerides.

SURGICAL PROCEDURES More frightening are treatment procedures which attempt to bypass the problem by surgery. A jejuno-ileal bypass is an operation in which part of the small intestine is inactivated so that food cannot be absorbed to the same extent. Normally performed in serious inflammatory diseases and cancer of the bowel, the bypass surgery has been performed for extreme obesity for the last twenty years. Its side effects have been extensively studied. Among the problems reported is psychological adjustment. In one follow-up study[11] thirty-two out of forty people experienced distinct crises associated with weight loss. These include, not surprisingly, problems about self-assertion, loss of identity and loss of boundaries. Another researcher reports[12] persistent overestimation of body size by female subjects two years after their operations after an average weight loss of 100–112 pounds.

An even more direct mechanical approach is the surgical removal of fat cells. In one experiment,[13] three patients were placed on reducing diets and when "normal" weight was achieved 47–60 percent of "excess fat cells" were removed. One patient suffered a thrombosis, one patient regained 81.4 pounds three years later and one patient keeps "a rigorous diet and regularly pursues a strenuous physical exercise program."

DIET THERAPY The diet remains the major treatment prescribed by doctors. Medical researchers investigate the effect of the relationship of various foods and offer their dieting programs accordingly. In comparison with the other treatments, dieting seems rather mild and harmless but it does not differ in principle from the more extreme drug or surgical therapies. It is as though the human body is the biological parallel of an automobile. Obesity is seen as a symptom of biological malfunction rather like a car's excess gas consumption. The human meanings of fat and thin and the social consequences and causes of compulsive eating have no place in this concept.

Although it is not my purpose to criticize those practititioners who are committed to human welfare, it is important to note that the medical profession as a whole has an unfortunate history of direct involvement with the oppression of women in our society. The work of Barbara Ehrenreich and

Deirdre English[14] has shown that the medical profession was established in the United States in the face of opposition from dedicated and informed lay healers, the majority of whom were women. Recently, women's health groups—most notably the Boston Women's Health Book Collective[15]— have rethought medical issues from a feminist perspective and have been engaged in sharing and disseminating the kind of information women need to know about their bodies. The activities of some women's groups have met with opposition from the authorities. In one case, women involved in a self-help group in California[16] were prosecuted (albeit unsuccessfully) for illegal entry of the vagina.

What is distressing about the current medical perspective is its hegemony in such areas as compulsive eating where the root causes and problems have essential social aspects that must be understood for there to be effective treatment and interventions. Even overweight diabetic women can be compulsive eaters and this problem needs to be addressed in conjunction with medical issues.

In the last decade we have seen a significant and increasing turn toward science and medicine to solve problems that are socially and economically based. Medicine is presented as the healer and science as the truth. A new religion reigns—the ideology of science.[17] This new ideology proposes that science is neutral and value free. White-coated men and women work away in laboratories seeking truth and progress. Medical researchers are not only truth seekers but humane too, since their work directly relates to human health. Few ask who funds the research and sets the priorities. Instead, the public are asked to embrace new technological fixes for human behavior issues.

A glance through the medical journals reveals this attitude in another area. Typically, you see a picture of a distraught woman in her forties slumped over a table in a messy kitchen. The advertisement reads in bold type, "X drug will help relieve the tension so she can cope better." In smaller print the advertisement mentions the familiar situation of the depressed menopausal woman who feels lifeless, with no energy now that her children have flown the nest. It recommends X psychotropic drug to reduce the anxiety. Doctors, who are frequently male, overworked, untrained to see the social issues that have produced distress in their women patients and unlikely to face this kind of distress themselves, recommend tranquilizers and psycho-active drugs to lift the spirits of these women so that they can function well enough again to clean up their own kitchens and not be a nuisance to anyone. The underlying social cause of distress is not dealt with. Medication is offered, the women are drugged.

Compulsive eating is an individual protest against the inequality of the sexes. As such, medical interventions as detailed here are not part of a solution but are part of the problem. The situation requires a major reorientation of medical and scientific education, organization and practice based on the demands of the women's health movement.

Notes

Preface

1. See chapter on medical issues. Analytic psychotherapy views eating behavior as a symptom that will dissolve when the true trauma has been resolved. It has not had any spectacular success in treating the symptom even in those cases where the person seeking therapy has come wanting to focus on compulsive eating as *the* problem.

2. See, for example:
Science for People 34 (winter 1976–7). A discussion on the relationship between food supplies, the politics of world agriculture and the exploitation of the resources of the Third World. Available from the British Society of Social Responsibility in Science, 9 Poland Street, London W.1, England.
   Science for the People 7 (March 1975).

3. In this case it will be important that therapists be extremely sensitive to their client's eating behavior and provide a place for her to feel accepted while she is self-rejecting because of the compulsive eating. It will also be important to look for transference issues both in group work and individual sessions.

Introduction

1. See, for example:
G. Bychowski, "Neurotic Obesity," *The Psychology of Obesity,* ed. N. Kiell (Springfield, Illinois, 1973).
Ludwig Bingswanger, "The Case of Ellen West," *Existence,* ed. Rollo May (New York, 1958).

2. William Ryan, *Blame the Victim* (New York, 1971). This book shows how we come to blame the victims of oppression rather than its perpetrators.

3. Dorothy Griffiths and Esther Saraga, "Sex Differences in a Sexist Society." Paper read at the International Conference on Sex-role Stereotyping, British Psychological Society, Cardiff, Wales, July 1977.

4. John Berger et al., *Ways of Seeing* (London, 1972), p. 47.

5. Simone de Beauvoir, *The Second Sex* (London, 1968).

6. For discussion on this see:
Juliet Mitchell, *Psychoanalysis and Feminism* (New York, 1974). Phyllis Chesler, *Women and Madness* (New York, 1972).

7. D. Brunet and I. Lezine, "I primi anni del bambino." Cited in Elena Gianini Belotti, *Little Girls* (London, 1975), pp. 32–4. While this study took place in Europe it does not rule out its relevance in the American context. The book in which it is extensively quoted is one of the most thoughtful descriptions of the socialization of young girls and the significance of the early sex-linked feeding relationship.

8. Margaret Atwood, *Lady Oracle* (London, 1977), p. 88.

What Is Thin About for the Compulsive Eater?

1. Sharon Rosenburg and Joan Weiner, *The Illustrated Hassle-Free Make Your Own Clothes Book* (San Francisco, 1971).

2. This is an Eastern European Jewish custom meant to bring color to the cheeks.

The Experience of Hunger for the Compulsive Eater

1. The diet industry is extremely profitable. For financial statistics see:
Natalie Allon, "The Stigma of Overweight in Everyday Life." John E. Fogarty International Center for Advanced Study in the Health Sciences. Vol. II, part II. National Institute of Health, Bethesda, Md. Edited by George A. Bray. DHEW publication. U.S. Govt. printing office. October 1–3, 1973, pp. 83–102.

2. Diet organizations will not release figures on recidivism. However, various sources put it at 95 percent. See Aldebaran, "Fat Liberation—A Luxury," *State and Mind* 5 (June–July 1977): 34.

3. Stanley Schachter, "Obesity and Eating," *Science* 161 (1968): 751.

4. For a discussion of this see:
A. J. Stunkard and H. M. McClaren, "The Results of Treatment for Obesity," *Archives of Internal Medicine* 103 (1959): 79.
Stanley Schachter, "Some Extraordinary Facts About Obese Humans and Rats," *American Psychologist* 23 (1971): 129.
Stanley Schachter, "Obesity and Eating," *Science* 161 (1968): 751.

5. Carol Bloom, "Training Manual for the Treatment of Compulsive Eating and Fat." Master's thesis, State University of New York at Stony Brook (1976).

Self-Starvation—Anorexia Nervosa

1. Mara Selvini Palazzoli, *Self Starvation* (London, 1974), pp. 24–5.

2. For useful discussions on anorexia nervosa see:
Rosie Parker and Sarah Mauger, "Self Starvation," *Spare Rib* 28 (1976).
Marlene Boskind-Lodahl, "Cinderella's Stepsisters: A

Feminist Perspective on Anorexia Nervosa and Bulimia,"
Signs 2 (winter, 1976): 342–56.
Mara Selvini Palazzoli, *Self Starvation* (London, 1974).
Hilde Bruch, *Eating Disorders* (New York, 1973).
Peter Dally, *Anorexia Nervosa* (London, 1969).
Anna Freud, "The Psychoanalytic Study of Infantile
Feeding Disturbances," *The Psychoanalytic Study of the
Child II* (London, 1946).

3. Parker and Mauger, "Self Starvation."

4. Palazzoli, *Self Starvation*, pp. 224–52.

5. Bruch, *Eating Disorders*, p. 88.

6. Dally, *Anorexia Nervosa*, pp. 93–4.

Medical Issues

1. J. L. Hirsch and J. Knittle, "Cellularity of Obese and
Nonobese Adipose Tissue," *Federation Proceedings of
the American Society for Experimental Biology* 29
(1970): 1516.

2. W. B. Kannel and T. Gordon, "Some Determinants of
Obesity and Its Impact as a Cardiovascular Risk Factor,"
in *Recent Advances in Obesity Research,* ed. Alan
Howard (London, 1975), p. 14. (Hereafter cited as *Recent
Advances.*)

3. H. E. Dugdale and P. R. Payne, "The Pattern of
Lean and Fat Deposition in Adults," *Nature* 266 (March,
1977): 349.

4. H. Keen, "The Incomplete Story of Obesity and
Diabetes," in Howard, *Recent Advances.*

5. R. C. Atkins, *Dr. Atkins' Diet Revolution* (New
York, 1972).

6. L. J. Herberg, K. B. J. Franklin and D. N. Stephens,
"The Hypothalamic 'Set Point' in Experimental Obesity,"
in Howard, *Recent Advances.*

7. Hilde Bruch, *Eating Disorders* (New York, 1973), p. 36.

8. Michael Schwartz and Joseph Schwartz, "No Evidence for Heritability of Social Attitudes," *Nature* 255: 429.

9. A. Cooke et al., "The New Synthesis Is an Old Story," *New Scientist* 70 (1976).

10. Ibid.

11. E. Espmark, "Psychological Adjustment Before and After Bypass Surgery for Extreme Obesity, a Preliminary Report," in Howard, *Recent Advances,* p. 242.

12. R. C. Kalucy et al., "Self Reports of Estimated Body Widths in Female Obese Subjects with Major Fat Loss Following Ileo-jejunal Bypass Surgery," in Howard, *Recent Advances,* p. 331.

13. J. G. Kral and L. V. Sjorstrom, "Surgical Reduction of Adipose Tissue Hypercellularity," in Howard, *Recent Advances,* p. 327.

14. Barbara Ehrenreich and Deirdre English, *Witches, Midwives and Nurses* (New York, 1973).

15. The Boston Women's Health Collective, *Our Bodies, Ourselves* (New York, 1973).

16. *People v. Carolyn Aurillia Downer* LAMC 31426942 (1972).

17. R. M. Young, "Science Is Social Relations," *Radical Science Journal* 5 (1977): 65.

Further Reading

Allon, Natalie, "Group Dieting Interaction." Unpublished doctoral dissertation, Brandeis University, Waltham, Mass. (1972).

Belotti, Elena Gianini, *Little Girls* (London, 1975).

Bloom, Carol, "Training Manual for the Treatment of Compulsive Eating and Fat." Master's thesis, State University of New York at Stony Brook (1976).

Boston Women's Health Book Collective, *Our Bodies, Ourselves* (New York, 1971).

Bruch, Hilde, *Eating Disorders* (New York, 1973).

Bernard, Jessie, *The Future of Motherhood* (New York, 1975).

Chesler, Phyllis, *Women and Madness* (New York, 1972).

de Beauvoir, Simone, *The Second Sex* (London, 1968).

Deutch, Helene, *The Psychology of Women,* vols. I & II (New York, 1973).

Donovan, Lynn, *The Anti Diet* (New York, 1971).

Ehrenreich, Barbara and English, Deirdre, *Witches, Midwives and Nurses* (New York, 1973).

Figes, Eva, *Patriarchal Attitudes* (Greenwich, Conn., 1970).

Friday, Nancy, *My Mother, My Self: The Daughter's Search for Identity* (New York, 1977).

Gerrard, Don, *One Bowl* (New York, 1974).

Kneill, N., ed., *The Psychology of Obesity* (Springfield, Ill., 1973).

Maccoby, Eleanor Emmons and Jacklin, Carol Nagy, *The Psychology of Sex Differences* (Stanford, Ca., 1974).

Mahler, Margaret, et al., *The Psychological Birth of the Human Infant* (New York, 1976).

McBride, Angela Barron, *The Growth and Development of Mothers* (New York, 1973).

McBride, Angela Barron, *Living with Contradictions: A Married Feminist* (New York, 1977).

Mitchell, Juliet, *Psychoanalysis and Feminism* (New York, 1974).

Pearson, Leonard and Lillian, *The Psychologist's Eat Anything Diet* (New York, 1973).

Reich, Wilhelm, *The Sexual Revolution* (New York, 1969).

Rosaldo, Michele Zimbalist and Lamphere, Louise, eds. *Women, Culture and Society* (Stanford, Ca., 1974).

Rubin, Theodore Issac, *Forever Thin* (New York, 1970).

Rich, Adrienne, *Of Women Born: Motherhood as Experience and Institution* (New York, 1976).

Sager, Clifford J. and Kaplan, Helen Singer, eds., *Progress in Group and Family Therapy* (New York, 1972).

Strouse, Jean, ed., *Women and Analysis* (New York, 1974).

Thompson, Clara, "Penis Envy in Women," *Psychiatry* 6 (1943).

Williams, Elizabeth Friar, *Notes of a Feminist Therapist* (New York, 1977).

Winnicot, D. W., *Mother and Child: A Primer of First Relationships* (New York, 1957).

Zaretsky, Eli, *Capitalism, the Family and Personal Life* (London, 1976).